Study Guide to Accompany
Berger and Williams
Fundamentals of Nursing
Collaborating for Optimal Health

Compiled By

Mary Anne Gauthier, RN, EdD
Northeastern University
Boston, Massachusetts

Barbara Kelley, RN, EdD
Northeastern University
Boston, Massachusetts

Joan Garity, RN, EdD
University of Massachusetts–Boston
Boston, Massachusetts

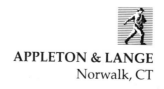

APPLETON & LANGE
Norwalk, CT

Copyright © 1993 by Appleton & Lange
Simon & Schuster Business and Professional Group

0-8385-2788-4

93 94 95 96 97 / 10 9 8 7 6 5 4 3 2 1

Prentice Hall International (UK) Limited, *London*
Prentice Hall of Australia Pty. Limited, *Sydney*
Prentice Hall Canada, Inc., *Toronto*
Prentice Hall Hispanoamericana, S.A., *Mexico*
Prentice Hall India Private Limited, *New Delhi*
Prentice Hall of Japan, Inc., *Tokyo*
Simon & Schuster Asia Pte. Ltd., *Singapore*
Editora Prentice Hall do Brasil Ltda., *Rio de Janeiro*
Prentice Hall, *Englewood Cliffs, New Jersey*

Production: P.S. Associates, Inc.
              Brookline, Massachusetts

PRINTED IN THE UNITED STATES OF AMERICA

CONTRIBUTORS

Constance J. Adams, RN, MPH, DrPH
Associate Dean for Nursing Practice
Indiana University School of Nursing
Assistant Director for Nursing Practice
Indiana University Hospitals
Indianapolis, Indiana

Donna J. Algase, RN, PhD
Assistant Professor of Nursing and
Assistant Research Scientist
University of Michigan School of Nursing
Division of Acute, Critical, and Long-term
Care Programs
Ann Arbor, Michigan

Christine Alster, RN, EdD
Associate Professor
College of Nursing
University of Massachusetts - Boston
Boston, Massachusetts

Ann N. Baker, RN-CS, PhD
Clinical Director, Critical Care and Psychiatric
Nursing
and Adjunct Assistant Professor, Nursing
School of Nursing
Medical College of Ohio
Toledo, Ohio

Karen J. Berger, RN, MS, EdD(c)
Doctoral Candidate, University of San Diego
San Diego, California
Formerly, Professor and Assistant Director,
Department of Nursing Education
Grossmont College, El Cajon, California
and Adjunct Instructor of Nursing
Pepperdine University, Vista Campus,
Vista, California

Ellen W. Bernal, PhD
Hospital Ethicist
St. Vincent Medical Center
Toledo, Ohio

Keith E. Boles, PhD
Associate Professor, Health Services Management
University of Missouri, Columbia
Columbia, Missouri

Nancy L. Bradley, RN, MEd
Assistant Professor of Nursing
Coordinator, Sophomore Nursing
School of Nursing
Kent State University
Kent, Ohio

Verna Benner Carson, RN, PhD
Assistant Professor, Psychiatric/Community Health
Nursing
School of Nursing
University of Maryland
Baltimore, Maryland

Deanna F. Cedargren, RN, PhD
Associate Professor, Nursing
School of Nursing
Medical College of Ohio
Toledo, Ohio

Mary Jo Clark, RN, PhD
Assistant Professor
Philip Y. Hahn School of Nursing
University of San Diego
San Diego, California

Joseph K. Davie, RN, MSN
Dean, School of Nursing
The Long Island College Hospital
Brooklyn, New York
Member, Diagnosis Review Committee
North American Nursing Diagnosis Association

Joan Garity, RN, EdD
Assistant Professor
College of Nursing
University of Massachusetts - Boston
Boston, Massachusetts

Mary Anne Gauthier, RN, EdD
Assistant Professor
College of Nursing
Northeastern University
Boston, Massachusetts

Delores J. Harkins, RNC, MS
Associate Professor of Nursing
School of Nursing
Medical College of Ohio
Toledo, Ohio

Lanis L. Hicks, PhD
Associate Professor, Health Services Management
University of Missouri, Columbia
Columbia, Missouri

Linda M. Hollinger, RN, PhD
Assistant Chairperson for Education
and Associate Professor
College of Nursing
Rush University
Chicago, Illinois

Julie E. Johnson, RN, PhD
Associate Dean and Associate Professor
College of Nursing
Montana State University
Bozeman, Montana

Barbara Kelley, RN, EdD
Assistant Professor
College of Nursing
Northeastern University
Boston, Massachusetts

Judith A. Lewis, RNC, PhD
Assistant Professor
Graduate Program in Nursing
MGH Institute of Health Professions
Boston, Massachusetts

Ruth Ludwick, RN, MSN
Assistant Professor
School of Nursing
Kent State University
Kent, Ohio

Susan L. MacLean, RN, PhD
College of Nursing
Rush University
Chicago, Illinois

Sherry L. Merrow, RN, EdD
Associate Professor
College of Nursing
University of Massachusetts - Boston
Boston, Massachusetts

Georgine Redmond, RN, EdD
Associate Professor and
Assistant Dean, Student Affairs
School of Nursing
George Mason University
Fairfax, Virginia

Connie Vaughn Roush, RN, MSN
Formerly, Assistant Professor
Point Loma Nazarene College
San Diego, California

Barbara Sarter, RN, FNP, FAAN, PhD
Associate Professor
Department of Nursing
University of Southern California
Los Angeles, California

Patricia F. Schmidt, RN, EdD
Associate Professor
Nursing Education Department
Palomar College
San Marcos, California

Carol A. Sedlak, RN, MSN, CCRN, ONC
Associate Professor
School of Nursing
Kent State University
Kent, Ohio

Jane C. Swart, RN, PhD
Dean and Professor
School of Nursing
Wright State University, Miami Valley
Dayton, Ohio

Donna F. Ver Steeg, RN, FAAN, PhD
Maternal-Child Health/Primary Ambulatory Care
Section
School of Nursing
University of California, Los Angeles
Los Angeles, California

Marilyn Brinkman Williams, RN, MSN
Professor, Department of Nursing Education
Grossmont College
El Cajon, California

CONTENTS

UNIT SEVEN: SCIENTIFIC AND PHILOSOPHICAL FOUNDATIONS OF NURSING PRACTICE

UNIT EIGHT: NURSING AND HEALTH CARE AS BUSINESS

PREFACE

This *Study Guide* is designed to accompany *Fundamentals of Nursing: Collaborating for Optimal Health*, by Karen J. Berger and Marilyn Brinkman Williams. To facilitate use, each chapter in the textbook has a corresponding chapter in the *Study Guide*. A variety of exercises are presented to assist you in recall and comprehension of essential knowledge and in analysis and application of that knowledge to clinical situations.

Each chapter of the *Study Guide* follows a standard organization.

Behavioral Objectives present essential content of the chapter in terms of expected learning outcomes.

Key Terms list terms from the chapter that you should understand and be able to define.

Review Questions highlight important chapter content. Emphasis is placed on application of content to clinical situations. You can use these questions to learn or review essential chapter content. Answers to review questions are found in the Answer Key at the back of the *Study Guide*, along with the page in the textbook on which the respective content appears.

Enrichment Activities are designed to be pursued, either alone or with a few other students, outside the classroom or clinical assignment. These activities are not greatly time consuming and are meant to enhance your understanding of important concepts in the textbook.

Self-Examination Questions offer an opportunity for you to assess your knowledge following the completion of study. Various testing strategies are used, including short answer, fill-in, true/false, matching, and multiple-choice questions. Answers are provided at the back of the *Study Guide*.

We hope that you will find this *Study Guide* both useful and enjoyable and welcome your comments.

CHAPTER 1

The Professional Nurse

■ BEHAVIORAL OBJECTIVES

After studying this chapter, you should be able to:

1. Define nursing according to the *ANA Social Policy Statement* and the models of caring, collaboration, and professionalism.

2. Describe the current role of the nurse in health care delivery.

3. Describe the typical nurse profile in the United States and Canada. Discuss trends influencing changes in these profiles.

4. Describe educational programs for generalist or specialist nursing practice.

5. Identify three credentialing mechanisms that are important to the education and practice of the nurse.

6. Describe major practice settings for nurses.

7. Discuss the roles of the nurse as caregiver, advocate, health care team member, manager, and decision-maker.

8. Describe the emerging role and functions of the nurse as entrepreneur.

9. Discuss ways in which the nurse collaborates with others to achieve optimal client health.

■ KEY TERMS

accreditation
case management
case nursing

certification
certified nurse-midwife
clinical nurse specialist

collaboration
credentialing
functional nursing

licensed practical
(vocational) nurse
licensure
nurse anesthetist

nurse practitioner
nursing
primary care

primary nursing
registered nurse
team nursing

■ REVIEW QUESTIONS

1. List four characteristics of successful nurses as perceived by clients, colleagues, and peers.

2. Name two trends influencing the typical nurse profile in the United States.

3. Identify three credentialing mechanisms that influence the education and practice of nurses.

4. Match the terms in column A with the correct descriptions in column B.

<u>A</u>

_____ (1) ANA *Social Policy Statement*

_____ (2) nursing as caring

_____ (3) nursing as collaboration

_____ (4) nursing as professionalism

<u>B</u>

a. transition based on mutual trust and mutual respect that facilitates independence in meeting health care needs

b. the identification and treatment of human responses to health problems

c. addressing matters of concern and significance to society using a specific body of knowledge and a self-enforced code of ethics

d. selecting caring behaviors and constructs by determining the meaning of caring for the one cared for

5. Name at least 10 ethnocaring concepts.

6. List five carative factors.

7. State the four minimal qualifications for professional status.

8. Match the terms in column A with the correct descriptions in column B.

A	B
_____ (1) planning	a. exercising power through evaluation and corrective measures to ensure achievement of plans
_____ (2) leading	b. coordinating integration of individual efforts and resources to bring about group efficiency and effectiveness
_____ (3) organizing	c. making decisions about what needs to be done and what will be done
_____ (4) controlling	d. influencing the behavior of workers to get them to do what needs to be done

9.   Describe three of the models of nursing care.

10.   List three major practice settings for nurses.

■ ENRICHMENT ACTIVITIES

1.   Ask four persons in your community who represent different ages and educational backgrounds to describe their views of the nurse. Meet with several of your colleagues to compare findings and determine whether the public image of the nurse differs by age or educational background of your respondents.

2.   Look for articles in popular magazines or watch television shows about nurses. How are nurses portrayed in the mass media? List the major kinds of activities in which nurses are involved. Describe how nurses interact with clients and other health care providers in the magazine articles or TV shows. How do the activities and behaviors of nurses in the media compare to those you've learned from your textbook or class discussions?

3.   Seek out two nursing students who are in nursing education programs that are at a different level than yours. For example, if you are enrolled in an associate degree nursing program, seek out students from diploma or baccalaureate nursing programs. Discuss reasons why they selected the programs they did. Share your reasons. Explore how your classes and learning experiences are different and how they are similar.

4.   Seek out three students in other health professions. Ask them about the major purpose and the common activities of the field they are studying. Discuss with them how you and they see themselves working as part of a health care team in the future.

5.   Talk to someone you know who has recently spent time in a hospital. Make a list of those things that person felt most positive about during the experience and those things the person liked least. Think about the implications for nurses of these likes and dislikes.

■ SELF-EXAMINATION QUESTIONS

1.   The ANA Social Policy Statement defines nursing as: _____

_____.

2. Match the theorists in column A with the appropriate concepts in column B.

<table>
<tr><td colspan="2" align="center"><u>A</u></td><td colspan="2"><u>B</u></td></tr>
<tr><td>_____</td><td>(1) Watson</td><td>a.</td><td>mutual interaction</td></tr>
<tr><td>_____</td><td>(2) Williamson</td><td>b.</td><td>transaction between nurse and client</td></tr>
<tr><td>_____</td><td>(3) Gaut</td><td>c.</td><td>carative factors</td></tr>
<tr><td>_____</td><td>(4) Kalisch</td><td>d.</td><td>purposeful intent</td></tr>
<tr><td>_____</td><td>(5) Paterson and Zderad</td><td>c.</td><td>ethnocaring concepts</td></tr>
<tr><td>_____</td><td>(6) Leininger</td><td>f.</td><td>nursing image</td></tr>
</table>

3. Collaborative transactions are most effective when based on: _____

    _____.

4. List at least four sites other than hospitals in which nursing is practiced.

5. Two levels of credentialing are _____ and _____.

6. List four types of educational programs whose graduates sit for the NCLEX examination for registered nurse licensure.

CHAPTER 2

Nursing as a Profession

■ **BEHAVIORAL OBJECTIVES**

After studying this chapter, you should be able to:

1. Identify at least four characteristics of a profession.

2. Discuss the significance of professionalism to collaborative, collegial practice in health care.

3. Discuss the development of nursing from pre-Christian times to the present.

4. Identify at least six persons who have made significant contributions to nursing.

5. Name at least three professional nursing organizations and identify a major contribution each has made to the development of nursing as a profession.

6. Identify four role problems faced by nurses in today's health care system.

7. Describe at least three rights and three responsibilities of nurses.

8. List five current socio-political, economic, or professional trends and describe their influence on nursing and collaborative health care practice.

9. Discuss strategies by which nurses can develop their power bases to achieve a preferred future for nursing.

10. Discuss the significance of collaboration in health care practice for health care clients and the discipline of nursing.

■ **KEY TERMS**

accountability
American Academy of Nursing
American Association of Colleges
   of Nursing
American Nurses' Association
applied science
autonomy
body of knowledge
Canadian Nurses' Association

control
ethics
International Council of Nurses
National Black Nurses'
   Association
National Federation for Specialty
   Nursing Organizations
National League for Nursing

National Student Nurses'
   Association
paternalism
profession
professional values
role transition
sexism
Sigma Theta Tau

■ **REVIEW QUESTIONS**

1. List two characteristics of any profession.

2. Match the term in column A with the description in column B.

       <u>A</u>   <u>B</u>

_____ (1) Florence   a. fought to change care for the mentally ill
              Nightingale
                                          b. developed collegiate education programs for
_____ (2) Dorothea Dix   nurses

_____ (3) Lillian Wald   c. identified teaching as a critical component of
                                              nursing
_____ (4) Mary Adelaide
              Nutting   d. established the American Red Cross

_____ (5) Clara Barton   e. wrote the first nursing text

_____ (6) Isabel Robb   f. pioneered community health nursing

3. Name two roles problems encountered by nurses in today's health care system.

4.   Match the groups in column A with the appropriate description in column B.

<u>A</u>

_____ (1) National League for Nursing

_____ (2) American Nurses' Association

_____ (3) American Association of Colleges of Nursing

_____ (4) American Academy of Nursing

_____ (5) Canadian Nurses' Association

_____ (6) International Council of Nurses

_____ (7) Sigma Theta Tau

_____ (8) National Student Nurses' Association

<u>B</u>

a.   provides a forum for deans of schools of nursing

b.   international honor society for nursing

c.   U.S. federation of state nursing associations

d.   federation of territorial and provincial nurses' associations

e.   limited to nurses who've made significant contributions to nursing research or practice

f.   involves students in issues of education at the state level

g.   sets educational standards for schools of nursing

h.   promotes communication among nurses throughout the world

5.   Name three rights and three responsibilities of nurses.

6.   Identify three of the five current social trends influencing nursing and collaborative health practice.

7. Distinguish differences between a job and a profession.

8. Name two strategies for achieving a preferred future for nursing.

9. Define autonomy, control, and accountability in practice.

10. Describe the effects of the feminist movement on the profession of nursing.

■ ENRICHMENT ACTIVITIES

1. Ask several people (relatives, neighbors) in your community to name five major professions. Then indicate on a scale of 1 (low) to 10 (high) the extent to which they trust those professions to be sincerely committed to helping people in need. Was nursing named? If it was named, did it receive higher or lower ratings than other professions?

2. Talk with a student from another health care discipline. Determine whether he or she perceives that nursing and the practitioners in his or her discipline currently collaborate in practice. List ways in which different health care providers need to collaborate to improve client care and outcomes.

3. Talk with two or three working nurses. Ask them to describe problems they encountered as new graduates entering a first position. Can you identify any similarities, differences, or patterns in problems identified?

4. Talk with neighbors who have children in elementary or high school. Ask them if they would like to see their daughter or son choose nursing for their future career. Ask them to tell you why they answered as they did. What do the reasons offered tell you about nursing's public image? Do people feel differently about nursing as a career for sons or daughters?

5.   Scan local newspapers for about two weeks for stories related to health care costs. Do any of the stories mention nursing? If so, in what context? List the issues that are included in the stories. Talk with a few of your classmates to discuss what nursing could do to have an impact on the issues related to health care costs.

■ **SELF EXAMINATION QUESTIONS**

1.   List four characteristics of a profession. Describe one achievement nursing has had related to each characteristic.

2.   The "dark age of nursing" ended in the:
      A. 1600s.
      B. 1700s.
      C. 1800s.
      D. 1900s.

3.   Match the names in column A with the appropriate descriptions in column B.

<u>A</u>

_____ (1) Dorothea Lynde Dix

_____ (2) Clara Barton

_____ (3) Lillian Wald

_____ (4) Annie Goodrich

_____ (5) Melinda Ann Richards

<u>B</u>

a. cared for soldiers during Civil War

b. community health nurse who developed nursing settlements

c. superintendent of female nurses of Union Army

d. first trained nurse in the United States

e. leader in developing collegiate education for nurses

4.   Identify one socio-political, economic, or professional trend and describe its influence on nursing.

5. Match the terms in column A with the correct definitions in column B.

<u>A</u>   <u>B</u>

_____ (1) autonomy   a. basis for body of knowledge

_____ (2) collaboration   b. self-directed clinical practice

_____ (3) research   c. payment for nursing care

_____ (4) nursing diagnosis   d. component of nursing process that is outcome
                                                of client assessment
_____ (5) direct reimbursement
                                            e. working together

6. Identify five role problems faced by nurses in today's health care system.

CHAPTER 3

Legal Considerations

■ **BEHAVIORAL OBJECTIVES**

After studying this chapter, you should be able to:

1. Describe in general terms the functions of licensure for a profession.

2. Compare and contrast the Nurse Practice Act for the state in which your school is located to the more general discussion in the chapter.

3. Describe the principles of client rights within the health care system.

4. Describe the usefulness of collaboration among health care team members and with clients in preventing misunderstandings and lawsuits.

5. Describe the principles involved in a living will and durable power of attorney for health care for clients and health care professionals.

6. Discuss the role of accurate record-keeping as a nursing responsibility as demonstrated by completing examples of actual chart and incident report forms from your clinical facility.

7. List the resources available to nurses for advice regarding legal and/or ethical problems in general and in your current practice location.

8. List seven examples of actions by nurses that will result in discipline by their state licensing board.

9. Compare and contrast the collaborative responsibilities of health care professionals and clients in the delivery of health care.

■ KEY TERMS

accreditation
administrative regulations
assault
battery
civil law
common law
community/locality standards
constitutional law
criminal law
dependent functions
durable power of attorney
employment contract

expert witness
felony
good samaritan laws
incompetence
independent functions
informed consent
informed dissent
intentional tort
laws
licensure
living will
malpractice suit

misdemeanors
negligence
nurse practice act
protocol
reciprocity
respondeat superior
slow code
statutory law
sunset laws
sunshine laws
tort
unintentional tort

■ REVIEW QUESTIONS

1. List the four categories of law.

2. Match the terms in column A with the correct descriptions in column B.

A

_____ (1) constitutional law

_____ (2) statutory law

_____ (3) common law

_____ (4) administrative regulations

B

a. case law that establishes precedents for future decisions

b. regulations that guide the implementation of statutes

c. law enacted by the legislative arm of government at the federal, state, or local level

d. a system of fundamental laws that establishes the structure and powers of government and the rights of its citizens

3.   List four examples of nurses' actions that will result in discipline by the state licensing board.

4.   Identify the six components of a Nurse Practice Act.

5.   List the four circumstances a plaintiff must demonstrate to prevail in a malpractice suit against a health care professional.

6.   Medical licensure encompasses the right to practice any branch of medicine regardless of the experience of the practitioner. True or False?

7.   Name two resources available to nurses for advice regarding legal and/or ethical problems.

8.   List three examples of client rights.

9. Define licensure of a profession in general.

10. Identify four ways nurses can avoid negligent torts.

■ **ENRICHMENT ACTIVITIES**

1. Scan the daily newspapers and current news magazines for a few weeks for articles related to professional malpractice. What did the practitioner do that was considered malpractice? How was the incident uncovered? What legal authorities were involved--the licensing board or the local district attorney? What kind of action is contemplated against the accused? How long ago did the malpractice occur? What, if any is the position of the client against whom the malpractice occurred? If the professional involved is not a nurse, how does malpractice in this profession compare to malpractice in nursing? What are the common threads?

2. The next time you are in the library, select a nursing journal for the year and month of your birth and one for the year of your mother's birth. How do the articles compare to those in current journals? Is there coverage of legal issues? Are there other (e.g., ethical) discussions of how nurses are expected to act? In what ways is nursing depicted as the same or different from today? What is the relationship to clients? To other health care professionals? To the employer?

3. Talk to several nurses who have been in practice for a while. How do they view the legal responsibilities of nurses in relation to documenting nursing action? Do they feel it is important? Do their opinions differ? In what way?

■ **SELF-EXAMINATION QUESTIONS**

1. List four functions of licensure.

2. A legal document that gives a named person the right to make health care decisions for another person is called a _____.

3. Clients' rights within the health care system are based on the principle(s) of:
A. autonomy.
B. privacy
C. doing no harm.
D. A and B.

4. A law that protects the nurse who stops and helps out at the scene of an accident is called a _____.

5. Malpractice as the result of omission of an act is called _____. Malpractice resulting from

    commission of an act is called _____.

6. The signature of a witness on an informed consent form means that the witness:
    A. instructed the client as to the procedure.
    B. filed the form in the chart.
    C. saw the client sign the form.
    D. certifies that the client understands the procedure.

CHAPTER 4

Politics, Policy Making, and Nursing

■ **BEHAVIORAL OBJECTIVES**

After studying this chapter, you should be able to:

1. Describe the steps in the policy-making process.

2. Discuss the relevance of the policy-making process to the practice of professional nursing.

3. Discuss the responsibility of nurses in the policy-making process.

4. Discuss the strategies available to nurses to influence the outcome of the policy-making process.

5. Describe the modes of lobbying nurses can use to influence public policy.

6. List the "do's" and "don'ts" of successful lobbying.

7. Discuss the current and potential role of professional nursing organizations in the policy arena.

8. Identify governmental agencies that affect nursing practice.

9. Discuss ways in which nurses collaborate to effect political change.

■ **KEY TERMS**

agencies	change	commissions
appropriating legislation	coalition	expert power
authorizing legislation	coercive power	incremental change
boards	collective bargaining	legislative process
boycott	collective power	legitimate power

lobbying
personal power
policy
policy evaluation
policy implementation
policy-making

political action committee
politics
power
public policy
radical change

referent power
regulation
reward power
special interest group
testimony

■ REVIEW QUESTIONS

1. List the steps in the policy-making process.

2. Describe the role of the nurse in the policy-making process.

3. Name five strategies the nurse can use to influence the outcomes of the policy-making process.

4. Identify three lobbying methods available to the nurse that can influence public policy.

5. List three do's and three don'ts for successful lobbying of public officials.

6. Identify four levels of government that affect nursing practice.

7. Discuss the differences between politics and policy.

8. Why is the vote important in establishing public policy?

9. Briefly describe three sources of power.

10. Name three tools for influencing the electoral process.

■ **ENRICHMENT ACTIVITIES**

1. Name as many policy-makers as you can who represent the community or district in which you live:

    • Mayor

    • City council members

    • County council members or supervisors

    • Governor

    • State house and senate legislators

    • President

    • National house and senate legislators

    Can you state the positions of these individuals on any health-related issues? For example, what is the position of your mayor on anti-smoking ordinances?

2. Candidates for elective office run in defined legislative districts that vary according to level of government, whether municipal, county, state, or federal. Do you know the legislative districts in which you live? If not, call the Registrar of Voters in your community. Ask for copies of the legislative maps for your community for each level of government. Locate your districts on these maps, using the address you listed on your voter's registration. How close do you live to the lines that divide your district from other districts? What difference does this make when you and your neighbors vote?

3. The next time you are in the library, look for issues of the official publication of your state nurses' association. If you don't know its name, the reference librarian will help you. Are there any articles that refer to lobbying activities by your state nurses' association? What policy issues do these articles address? Do they name the lobbyists for the association?

4. Looking at the same publication, find articles that deal with coalitions between the state nurses' association and other organizations on particular political or health care issues. What issues are involved? Find a copy of a publication put out during a presidential or congressional campaign. Did your state nurses' association endorse any candidates? For what reasons?

■ **SELF-EXAMINATION QUESTIONS**

1. List the steps in the policy-making process.

2. One difference between laws and regulations is that laws are _____

    and regulations are _____.

3. True or false: In the legislature, committee chairs are always members of the party that holds the majority of seats in that chamber.

4. List at least five ways the nurse can lobby a legislator.

5. True or false: At public hearings, private citizens have the opportunity to listen to legislators express their opinions about why a particular bill should be supported or defeated.

6. True or false: After a bill becomes a law there is no longer any opportunity to exert influence regarding its provisions.

CHAPTER 5

Health and Illness

■ **BEHAVIORAL OBJECTIVES**

After studying this chapter, you should be able to:

1. Discuss why it is important to develop clear definitions of health and wellness, disease and illness.

2. Describe the role-performance, clinical, adaptive, and eudaimonistic models of health.

3. State the distinction between health and wellness.

4. Define optimal health.

5. List several health promotion measures.

6. State the distinctions among illness, disease, and deviance.

7. Discuss the concept of a health-illness continuum. Contrast 2 models of health continuua.

8. Discuss the ways in which theories of disease causation influence health behavior.

9. Give examples of primary, secondary, and tertiary measures for disease prevention.

10. Identify factors that may prevent clients from adopting positive health behaviors.

11. Outline the roles of both nurse and client when collaborating on health promotion and disease prevention.

■ KEY TERMS

adaptation	health-illness continuum	multiple-causation theory
at-risk role	health maintenance	optimal health
deviance	health promotion	primary prevention
disease	high-level wellness	role-modeling
disease prevention	holistic health	secondary prevention
etiology	informed dissent	tertiary prevention
eudaimonistic	maladaptation	wellness

■ REVIEW QUESTIONS

1. Provide brief definitions for health, wellness, disease and illness and describe why it is important for nurses to have clear definitions of these terms.

2. Name four factors that have a significant influence on a client's health.

3. List four roles of professional nurses that assist clients to improve their health.

4. Give an example of how a nurse promotes health through role-modeling.

5. Discuss the strengths and limitations of Brubaker's health-illness continuum.

6. Match the terms in column A with the correct descriptions in column B.

<u>A</u>   <u>B</u>

_____ (1) primary prevention   a. contact follow-up in cases of sexually transmitted disease

_____ (2) secondary prevention   b. providing information to the public on how to avoid sexually transmitted diseases

_____ (3) tertiary prevention   c. treatment of a person infected with syphilis

_____ (4) health promotion   d. engaging in exercise on a regular basis

7. List the five leading causes of death in the United States and identify a current health practice that is directed toward preventing each of these causes of death.

8. Explain how a nurse may incorporate all three levels of disease prevention in practice and give an example of each.

9. Mary Jones, a 34-year-old black woman, is married and has three children, ages 8, 9, and 12. She is seventy pounds overweight and has mild hypertension. Outline the role of the nurse and the client when collaborating on the client's goal to reduce weight and reduce her blood pressure.

10. After collaborating with Mary on her plan, you say good-bye in the waiting room, where Mary introduces you to two of her children, both boys. You notice that they too are quite overweight. In planning for a future appointment with Mary, what are some topics to include?

■ ENRICHMENT ACTIVITIES

1. Interview a person in stable health about his or her health status. Ask the person to rate his or her personal health on a scale from one to ten in the following areas: sleep and rest, exercise, nutrition, stress level, safety practices, and substance use. Make sure the person indicates the specifics on which the rating is based. Do you agree with the individual? Would your rating differ? What is the person's frame of reference--with whom does the person compare himself or herself? What is your frame of reference for rating the person?

2. Make a list of behaviors and practices that you believe are important for maintaining health and preventing disease for a person of your age. Does your list agree with authoritative lists found in health care literature? Which behaviors or practices do you incorporate into your own life? Are there any you ignore? What barriers prevent you from carrying out all of the activities you feel are important? Discuss your list with a friend. Do your lists agree? Are your practices similar? How about the things you do not practice? Are there any common barriers you perceive? How would an understanding of such barriers help you be more effective as a nurse?

3. As Chapter 5 indicates, people use various models of health to evaluate their own and others' conditions. It is important for nurses to understand these models in behavioral terms. Consider the following example and decide which models are shaping the client's and nurse's behavior.

    Bob, who works on the plant loading dock, reports to the employee health office nurse. He wants to return to work after a 2-week absence for a back injury. He says he has resumed his normal activities at home and is ready to return. He tells the nurse he has been helping his daughter move into a new apartment, which, he points out, involves the same kind of heavy lifting required by his job. The nurse asks Bob several questions about pain, and he admits that he continues to have pain in his leg, as he had after the injury occurred. The nurse examines Bob's posture, gait, and range of motion.

4. The mass media are a powerful source of images of health. The next time you watch television, pay particular attention to the commercials presented and categorize them as to the models of health they depict. How many of them seem to depict a clinical model of health? What kinds of products are promoted by associating them with the alleviation of symptoms of illness? Do any of the commercials seem to portray a eudaimonistic model of health? Do they seek to sell products by associating them with self-actualization?

■ SELF-EXAMINATION QUESTIONS

1. Definitions of health and illness:
    A. are similar among all cultures.
    B. refer primarily to physical condition.
    C. are fluid and vary over time and among groups.
    D. are consistent among health care providers.

2.   Match the descriptions of health in column A with the correct models in column B.

	A		B
_____	(1) the ability of a person to carry out expected functions		a. clinical model
_____	(2) the full expression of a person's potential		b. role performance model
_____	(3) the absense of disease or illness		c. adaptive model
_____	(4) the ability to respond successfully to challenging stimuli		d. eudaimonistic model

3.   True or false: Disease and illness are terms that refer to an observable disruption of structure or function in the person.

4.   Describe three aspects of the nurse's role in health promotion.

5.   True or false: When nurse and client collaborate to identify appropriate client behaviors to promote health, the nurse's knowledge carries more weight than the client's preferences.

6.   What is the appropriate nursing response to a client who declines to make life-style changes to prevent disease?

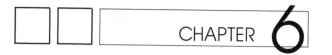

CHAPTER 6

Homeostasis, Homeodynamics, and Change

■ **BEHAVIORAL OBJECTIVES**

After studying this chapter, you should be able to:

1. Define human change.

2. Describe Lewin's three phases of change.

3. Give an example of each of the following patterns of change: maturational, situational, planned, unplanned, physiological, psychological, and social.

4. Define homeostasis and identify the two major homeostatic regulatory systems in the body.

5. Describe the effects of the two components of the autonomic nervous system on body systems and outline the "fight-or-flight" response.

6. Identify the components of a control mechanism, and give an example of a negative feedback system.

7. Compare homeostasis and adaptation and state their significance to health.

8. Define stressor and give examples of physiological, psychological, and social stressors.

9. Explain what is meant by stress as a transaction.

10. Identify the factors that regulate the cognitive appraisal of stress, and the physiological and psychological manifestations of stress.

11. Differentiate stress and crisis, and give examples of maturational and situational changes that may be experienced as crisis.

12. Identify six stress management techniques and describe how they work to neutralize stress.

13. Compare and contrast homeostatic and homeodynamic views of human change.

14. Describe the collaborative view of facilitating growth.

15. Discuss the nurse's role as participant in client change and the promotion of optimal health.

■ KEY TERMS

adaptation
alarm stage
anxiety
burnout
change
closed systems
cognitive appraisal
comparator
coping
crisis
defense mechanism
effector
exhaustion stage

fear
general adaptation syndrome
growth
hardiness
homeodynamics
homeostasis
maturational changes
maturational crises
mutual process
negative feedback
open systems
panic

planned change
positive feedback
receptor
resistance stage
response
situational changes
situational crises
stability
stress
stressor
system
unplanned change

■ REVIEW QUESTIONS

1. Provide a brief definition of change and describe why nurses need an understanding of change.

2. Describe change as a process. Using change as a process, describe the phases a person would need to pass through in order to stop smoking.

3. Mr. Edward, 76, enters the health care center with a broken wrist. Describe what the nurse needs to assess regarding Mr. Edward's response to the broken bone and the significance this change will have in his life.

4. List the factors that either enable or impede an individual who is dealing with stress.

5. Mr. James, a 60-year-old widower, is a shoe store manager. He states that he works twelve hours a day, can't sleep at night, and has lost his appetite. But he has gained twenty pounds lately because he eats candy bars as snacks. He appears tired and agitated, and his clothes are wrinkled and tight. He states that his father recently died. List the behavioral and emotional characteristics exhibited by Mr. James that indicate stress.

6. Describe how a nurse can use his or her knowledge of homeostasis and adaptation to stress to assist Mr. James.

7. Mrs. Powers accompanies her mother to the health clinic. The mother has Alzheimer's disease and currently has a urinary tract infection. While examining the mother, you notice that Mrs. Powers is very nervous. After the examination, Mrs. Powers bursts into tears and says that dealing with her mother is very difficult. You suggest that Mrs. Powers' mother wait in the examining room while you talk to Mrs. Powers. What would you assess to determine whether Mrs. Powers' coping patterns are effective in dealing with the care of her mother?

8. While talking with you, Mrs. Powers says she feels overwhelmed with caring for her mother, that there is a lot of tension in her home since her mother moved in, and that nothing seems to help and she has no other family members to turn to. What phase of crisis is Mrs. Powers in, and what are three possible outcomes for her?

9. Describe why nursing may be highly stressful.

10. Describe three stress management techniques for nurses.

■ ENRICHMENT ACTIVITIES

1. With a friend, complete the Social Readjustment Rating Scale. Discuss similarities and differences in the major life changes that you each have experienced in the last year. Compare and contrast the impact of similar life changes on your respective personal, family, and social lives.

2. Keep a diary for 1 week to identify daily activities and the feelings associated with these activities. At the end of the week, analyze the activities for those that could be described as hassles or uplifts. Review the diary for patterns of behavior (eg, patterns of sleeping, eating, studying, or work-related activities). Are these patterns the same throughout the week or do they change often? What seems to influence changes?

3. With a friend, review the list of possible stress-linked diseases and symptoms. Have either of you experienced any of these within the past month? Within the past year? What stressors were present when you experienced these symptoms? Does your physical response vary with different stressors?

4. Do you have particular physiological behavior patterns related to stress such as diarrhea or tightness in the neck or jaw? Do particular stressors affect your interactions with family/friends? Which ones? How does stress affect your ability to meet social obligations, such as work and school responsibilities?

5. Identify a person who knows you well and "cares" for you personally, and a person who is just an "acquaintance." These people may be friends, relatives, clergy, counselors, classmates, or teachers. How do you feel when these people are present?   Compare and contrast your relationships with these people in terms of your ability to communicate with them. Which one helps you feel more relaxed and less stressed? What factors seem to influence your feelings?

■ SELF-EXAMINATION QUESTIONS

1. The _____ and the _____ are the major homeostatic regulators in the body.

2. Match the physiologic effects in column A with the appropriate branches of the autonomic nervous system in column B (NOTE: the same answer may be used more than once in column A.)

<u>A</u>	<u>B</u>
_____ (1) increased rate and force of cardiac contraction	a. sympathetic
_____ (2) increased gastrointestinal motility	b. parasympathetic
_____ (3) bronchodilation	
_____ (4) peripheral vasoconstriction	

3. Excessive release of cortisol during the physiologic stress response may lead to which of the following deleterious effects?
   A. decrease in immune/inflammatory response
   B. heart palpitations
   C. stress ulcers
   D. A and C

4. Emotion-focused coping deals with a stressful experience by:
   A. resolving the situation causing the stress.
   B. avoiding the threat of the situation.
   C. reducing the tension of the situation.
   D. distracting the individual's attention away from the stressful experience.

5. It has been postulated that the mind and body communicate through:
   A. mind modulation.
   B. the limbic-hypothalamic system.
   C. the neuropeptide system.
   D. all of the above.

6. All of the following are true of homeodynamic principles *except*:
   A. they describe the nature and direction of human change.
   B. they are derived from nursing theory.
   C. they describe the behavior of human beings as wholes.
   D. they have the goal of maintaining stability.

7. All of the following encourage growth *except*:
   A. avoidance of conflict.
   B. spiritual compassion.
   C. energetic motivation.
   D. intellectual curiosity.

CHAPTER 7

Community Health

■ **BEHAVIORAL OBJECTIVES**

After studying this chapter, you should be able to:

1. Define the term "community" and identify several characteristics of a community.

2. Define the term "community health."

3. Distinguish among primary, secondary, and tertiary prevention.

4. List the members of the community health team.

5. Describe the components of the epidemiological triad.

6. List the steps of the epidemiological method.

7. Differentiate between mortality and morbidity, and between incidence and prevalence of disease.

8. Describe the chain of infection and state several ways that it can be broken.

9. Describe factors influencing the development of chronic diseases.

10. Discuss control strategies for communicable and chronic diseases and other community health problems.

11. State the importance of the concept of the community as client and describe the nurse's role in addressing the health needs of the community.

12. Discuss the role of the community health nurse as collaborator in community health nursing.

■ **KEY TERMS**

acquired immunity
active immunity
agent
carrier
chain of infection
clinical state
communicable disease
community
community health
community health nursing
direct transmission
discharge planning
epidemiological triad
epidemiology
health education
health promotion

host
immunity
immunization
incidence
indirect transmission
infectivity
morbidity rate
mortality rate
multiple causation
natural immunity
passive immunity
pathogenicity
portal of entry
portal of exit
preclinical state
preexposure stage

prevalence
primary prevention
rate
reservoir
resolution stage
risk
risk factor
screening
secondary prevention
target group
tertiary prevention
vaccine
vector
vehicle
virulence

■ **REVIEW QUESTIONS**

1.   Provide brief definitions of community health and public health. Describe why nurses need an understanding of community health.

2.   Identify the two major sectors of the health care delivery system in the United States and describe how they differ in terms of emphasis and focus of care.

3.   List two of the five categories of health promotion.

4. Mrs. Howe brings her three-month-old baby to the health center for a well-baby check-up. While Mrs. Howe is in the center, what strategies of health promotion should be employed?

5. Define epidemiology. Discuss why nurses need to understand the epidemiological triad model.

6. How does health promotion differ from disease prevention?

7. While you are taking Mrs. Dow's health history, she states that her mother died from a heart attack and her father died following a stroke. When collaborating with Mrs. Dow regarding health promotion and disease prevention, which strategies would you want to explore?

8. Mrs. Dow also states that she is currently being treated for diabetes. Describe the risk factors and the primary, secondary, and tertiary prevention strategies for diabetes mellitus.

9. Describe five roles of community health nurses.

10. Give a brief overview of the history of community health nursing.

■ **ENRICHMENT ACTIVITIES**

1. Communities are defined by common location, but also by common interests, needs, and collective action to meet them. Think of several groups of people you are familiar with--a church group, a campus association, a social club. In what sense are these groups communities? Can you think of a group of people that does not meet the criteria for a community? Do demographic age groups satisfy the criteria? How about a group of people who all have the same disease?

2. For one or more weeks, watch the local newspapers for articles related to accidents that involve traumatic injuries. What types of accidents are most frequently reported? Where did these accidents take place? What conditions--physical, social, and emotional--led to the accidents? Was prevention possible? Do any of the articles discuss community endeavors to prevent such accidents?

3. Read the obituary column of your newspaper for several days. What seems to be the most common cause of death reported? Were any deaths caused by preventable diseases? How old were the deceased persons when they died? Were any in the young adult period of life? Look for articles in the paper that discuss communicable disease in your community. Have there been any flare-ups of preventable infectious disease? What are the implications for nurses?

4. Call your local or county health department (the number can be found in the telephone book or can be obtained from information). Ask where and how to obtain immunizations for children. What kind of response did you get? Were the people you talked to helpful? Is there a community organization or network that assists people who desire to have their children immunized? What barriers might new people in your community encounter in getting their health needs met?

■ **SELF-EXAMINATION QUESTIONS**

1. Match the descriptions in column A with the definitions in column B.

<u>A</u>

_____ (1) group of people among whom there is some kind of bond and who interact to collectively solve common problems

_____ (2) interventions directed a resolving an acute health problem

_____ (3) interventions directed at maintaining and enhancing health

_____ (4) the study of factors that affect the occurrence and control of disease

_____ (5) the extent to which a given health problem occurs in a population

<u>B</u>

a. secondary prevention

b. community

c. morbidity

d. health promotion

e. health appraisal

f. epidemiology

2. Which of the following statements describes the difference between primary and tertiary prevention?
    A. Primary prevention refers to the prevention of disease complications; tertiary prevention refers to the prevention of secondary illnesses.
    B. Primary prevention refers to interventions before illness occurs; tertiary prevention refers to intervention after the acute phase of illness is resolved.
    C. Primary prevention refers to the strategies the health provider uses before the client has risk factors; tertiary prevention refers to the strategies applied after risk factors appear.

3. Name the three components of the epidemiological triad.

4. List four steps in the epidemiological method.

5. Which of the following statements describes the difference between incidence and prevalence?
    A. Incidence reflects the number of symptoms an individual has; prevalence is the number of people in the individual's family that have the same symptoms.
    B. Incidence reflects the number of people with the risk factors for a disease; prevalence reflects the number of people who are able to transmit the disease.
    C. Incidence reflects the number of new cases of a disease within a population; prevalence refers to the number of cases that exist at any point in time.

6. Direct care is an important function of the community health nurse. It includes all of the following *except*:
    A. teaching and counseling.
    B. coordinating the care of other health care professionals involved in assisting a client with multiple problems.
    C. role modeling.
    D. supervising the client's medications.

7. In what sense is a class of nursing students a community?

CHAPTER 8

Family Health

■ **BEHAVIORAL OBJECTIVES**

After studying this chapter, you should be able to:

1. Discuss the importance of the family in nursing.

2. Describe the relationship between the health of the individual and the health of the family.

3. Define the family in broad terms and as a health care unit.

4. List and describe various family forms.

5. Describe the structural and functional elements of the family.

6. List the eight stages of Duvall's family life cycle and discuss the developmental tasks involved in each stage.

7. Discuss crisis within a family and identify examples of developmental and situational crises experienced by families.

8. Describe the components of family assessment.

9. Discuss the role of family systems and self-care theories in collaborating with families.

10. Describe the nurse's role in comprehensive care of the family.

■ KEY TERMS

affective function
blended family
communal family
comprehensive family care
crisis
extended family
family
family assessment
family function

family of cycle
family of origin
family of procreation
family power structure
family structure
family value system
gay or lesbian family
maturational crisis
nuclear family

plural family
reproductive function
role
role complementarity
role set
singe-parent family
situational crisis
socialization and social
    placement function

■ REVIEW QUESTIONS

1. Provide a brief definition of family. Describe why it is important for nurses to recognize a variety of family norms.

2. Describe two approaches for understanding the family.

3. List the eight stages of Duvall's family life cycle.

4. Discuss the developmental tasks of each stage of Duvall's family life cycle.

5. Jane Edmonds, 17 years old, is pregnant. She comes to the health clinic in her fifth month of pregnancy. She has not told anyone of her pregnancy except her best girlfriend. She is afraid to tell her boyfriend (the father) or her mother. She has not seen her own father in two years. Describe which type of family crisis is occurring and the goal of crisis intervention.

6. What nursing interventions would be appropriate in working with this family?

7. In assessing the Edmonds family, the nurse needs to identify healthy aspects of the family and capitalize on these family strengths. What are the five characteristics of a healthy family?

8. Mrs. Scanlon is a new mother and is very anxious to fulfill her role of mother and wife. What family tasks related to health should the nurse review with Mrs. Scanlon?

9. The nurse tells Mrs. Scanlon that she would like to work with her regarding the health of her new family. What are the components of the family assessment?

10. How can the nurse facilitate Mrs. Scanlon's right to self-determination in health care?

■ ENRICHMENT ACTIVITIES

1. Compare your family with that of a friend. How do your two families differ as to form (nuclear, single-parent, etc.), developmental stage (married, no children; families with teenagers; etc.), structure and role allocation (who does the wage earning, childrearing, housekeeping, etc.), value system (family priorities), communication patterns (effectiveness in meeting members' needs), and power structure (decision-making authority)?

2. Contact a major church in your community. If possible, pick one that you are not familiar with. Talk to a knowledgeable person in the administrative office or to one of the clergy. Ask about activities the church provides to support family life, such as seminars in parenting, family counseling, outreach services for families, or other activities. How organized is this church in meeting family needs? Inquire about ways in which the church assists families to weather crises.

3. Call your local or county health department and ask about family services available in the community to help families in crisis. What kinds of problems do these community services respond to? Can these be related to the developmental cycle of the family? Does your community have an organized system for assisting families?

4. The next time you are in a bookstore, ask the salesperson to direct you to books that address family life in some way (for instance, books on childbearing, parenting and childrearing, marriage and divorce, caring for aging parents). How many different types of books are you able to find? Judging from the number of books available in the commercial market, do you think that family life is a matter of concern to the public?

■ SELF-EXAMINATION QUESTIONS

1. True or false: Two adults of the same sex who share an intimate relationship and life together are considered to be a family.

2. True or false: A task of a family with preschool children is to socialize their children and establish relationships with other families.

3. True or false: Separation and divorce may be experienced by the family as a maturational crisis.

4. True or false: In order to adequately assess the family, a nurse must listen carefully to the family's health concerns.

5. Two types of family crisis are _____ and _____.

6. Examples of family support networks include _____ and _____.

CHAPTER 9

Sociocultural and Spiritual Dimensions of Health

■ **BEHAVIORAL OBJECTIVES**

After studying this chapter, you should be able to:

1. Define the concept of culture.

2. Discuss the impact of culture on attitudes and habits.

3. Discuss ethnocentrism, and identify ways of becoming culturally sensitive.

4. State the relationship of cultural beliefs to health care practices.

5. Contrast the traditional and the modern health care cultures.

6. Discuss health beliefs and practices of several major cultural groups in the United States.

7. Discuss the relationship between the concepts of religion and spirituality.

8. Describe how spirituality, religion, and health interrelate with culture.

9. Discuss the relationship of religion to health practices.

10. Discuss the beliefs and practices of five prevalent religions in the United States.

11. Describe how intercultural collaboration between nurse and client promotes effective client care.

12. Define the principles of cultural relativism, cultural sensitivity, and transcultural reciprocity in nursing collaboration.

13. Identify the essential components of a cultural assessment.

14. Identify the nurse's role in planning care based on cultural differences.

■ **KEY TERMS**

acculturation	enculturation	religion
assimilation	ethnicity	social relationships
cultural conflict	ethnocentrism	social structure
cultural relativism	ideology	society
cultural sensitivity	minority culture	spirituality
culture	prejudice	stereotyping
culture shock	race	subculture
discrimination	racism	transcultural reciprocity
dominant culture		

■ **REVIEW QUESTIONS**

1. Define culture and describe why it is important for nurses to have an understanding of culture.

2. How is culture transmitted?

3. Describe your culture and how it influences your values, beliefs, and behaviors.

4. How do ethnicity and race differ?

5. How can nurses learn to become culturally sensitive? What role does cultural sensitivity play in healing and treating disease?

6. Using Table 9-1 in the text, discuss the health beliefs and practices described for a particular cultural group with a friend who is a member of that group. Does your friend agree or disagree with the generalizations?

7. Define spirituality. How does this differ from religion? What are the implications for nurse-client collaboration?

8. Mrs. Romonosky has recently moved to the neighborhood surrounding the health center. While doing a cultural assessment, the nurse discovers that Mrs. Romonosky is Ukrainian and that her religion is Eastern Orthodoxy. What questions regarding religion would the nurse find helpful in collaborating with this client's health needs?

9. Mohammand Salam, a Black Muslim, has been admitted to the hospital for major cardiac surgery. He is a diabetic. What implications does his religion have regarding his health care?

10. Martin Cohen is sitting with his father, who needs a kidney transplant. He is very concerned that his father, an Orthodox Jew, has refused this treatment. What are the nursing implications for collaboration with Mr. Cohen and his father? What resources in the hospital would you request?

■ ENRICHMENT ACTIVITIES

1. Diagram your family tree, going back as many generations as you can. Indicate national origin under the name of each member. Were any of your relatives born outside the United States or Canada?

2. Identify the holidays your family observes. Pick one and describe the rituals or ceremonies associated with it that you practice. Are there any special foods that you eat or clothes that you wear on that occasion? Why are these practices important to you and your family? List as many reasons as you can.

3.   Think of a friend who is of a different ethnic origin than yourself. What holidays does your friend observe? Are they different from your own? What rituals or ceremonies does he or she practice? Describe one. Have you ever participated with you friend in any of his or her holiday observances? How did you feel about the experience? List the feelings you had.

4.   What major ethnic groups are represented in the population of your community? What languages do they speak? List some attitudes or practices that individuals representing these ethnic populations might be expected to exhibit in relation to illness.

5.   Think about an experience you have had with being ill. List your symptoms. What did you do about those symptoms? Whom did you approach for advice? When you were sick, did anyone else help you? Who was that person? Did you use any remedies that might not be considered a part of scientific medicine? Have you ever experienced severe pain? How did you cope? Can you associate any of your behaviors during your experience with illness with your own ethnic background? Which ones?

■ SELF-EXAMINATION QUESTIONS

1.   List the characteristics of culture.

2.   Define enculturation.

3.   Define acculturation.

4.   List categories of attitudes that are influenced by culture.

5.   Define ethnocentrism.

6.   Define culture shock.

CHAPTER 10

The Client as an Individual

■ BEHAVIORAL OBJECTIVES

After studying this chapter, you should be able to:

1. Define the term "individuality."

2. Describe the phenomenologic view of perception.

3. Outline the five levels of basic human needs proposed by Maslow.

4. Describe five positive characteristics likely to be exhibited by a self-actualizing person.

5. Define the concept of identity and its component parts.

6. List six criteria useful for assessing the state of an individual's emotional health.

7. List the eight states of psychosocial development proposed by Erikson.

8. Outline the major tasks to be accomplished during each of the four transitional periods in one's life structure.

9. Explain how a collaborative approach to health care facilitates self-actualization.

■ KEY TERMS

body image	fixation	human needs
coping	gender	id
development	gender identity	identity
developmental task	gender role	individuality
ego	growth	integration

life structure
life-style
maturation
perceptions
perceptual field
personality

phenomenal self
regression
role performance
self
self-acceptance

self-concept
self-esteem
stress
stressors
superego

■ REVIEW QUESTIONS

1. Provide a brief definition of individuality. Discuss why it is important for nurses to understand clients as individuals.

2. Describe the basic human needs according to Maslow. Discuss why this concept is popular with nurses. How did Kalish modify Maslow's hierarchy of needs?

3. What are the five characteristics of a self-actualized person?

4. What are the components of self-concept?

5. John Smith, a 17-year-old high school senior is hospitalized after an automobile accident. He is paralyzed from the waist down. He is going to miss his final exams, senior prom, and the last baseball game of the year and of his high school career. What should the nurse anticipate as potential concerns of John while he is hospitalized?

6. According to Erikson, John Smith is in what stage of psychological development? What implications does this have for a nurse collaborating in John's care?

7. John Smith is in what stage of sexual development? What are the implications of his hospitalization?

8. John confides to the nurse that he possibly has been exposed to the HIV virus, through sexual activity. What preparations does the nurse need in order to address, accept, and understand a client's individual sexuality?

9. Margaret Lambert, a 62-year-old retired secretary, asks the nurse whether changes in sexuality occur with aging. How should the nurse respond to Miss Lambert?

10. Martha Jones, 47-years-old, is having her annual checkup. Identify the sexual issues that should be discussed with Mrs. Jones.

■ ENRICHMENT ACTIVITIES

1. Think about the way you live your life at present. What are the activities from which you derive the most satisfaction? Who are the people you see regularly? Which ones provide the greatest source of love, belonging, and esteem in your life? Are these individuals family members or friends? Think about their commitments and burdens--their job and family responsibilities, and so on. If you were to become hospitalized, what would be the impact on your relationship with them? How many would be available to give you support during the experience? What kind of support could you depend on them for? What influence would their support have on your sense of "who you are" during your hospital stay?

    What activities would you find most difficult to give up if you were hospitalized, even for a little while? Think about those activities. What about them makes them important to you? Do they allow you to perform a skill you are good at? Put you in contact with friends? Keep you from being bored? Give you a sense of accomplishment?

    How does sensitivity to issues such as these make you a better nurse?

2. Everyone has an identity, but identity has two aspects, a subjective aspect (self-concept) and an objective aspect (others' concepts of oneself). Think of the traits that you feel characterize you--appearance, attitudes, moods, values, goals, and what is important to you; how you look and feel; your talents; your habits (good and bad). Which traits are most typical of you? Write these down on a piece of paper, but do not put your name on it. Have three or four of your friends do the same thing. Trade your lists. Are you able to match the lists with the correct people? Do the self-perceptions of the people sharing this activity match with others' concepts of them? What are some of the implications for an individual's needs in instances where they do not match or where the match involves an undesirable trait?

3. Write a paragraph describing your present life structure using Levinson's concept of family, work, and leisure as the central elements in your description. How is your life structure different from what it was 5 years ago? Typically, school ranks very high among the priorities of nursing students. What aspects of your life did you minimize or give up to place emphasis on your education? What are the pros and cons of those sacrifices? How do you feel about the tradeoffs? Do you envision changes in your life structure after graduation? How would you describe the life-style that goes along with being a student? Hectic? Pressured? Stressful? Interesting? Confining? Exhilarating? Imagine being suddenly hospitalized for abdominal surgery that required you to miss two weeks of school. What would be the consequences for meeting your educational goals? On a piece of paper, list as many effects as you can that such an occurrence would have on your life.

■ SELF-EXAMINATION QUESTIONS

1. Define "individuality."

2. Self-actualization is:
    A. achieved by every individual during adulthood.
    B. a basic human need.
    C. never fully achieved by anyone.
    D. not an important human need.

3. Which of the following factors is not a component of self-concept?
    A. body image
    B. self-esteem
    C. self-actualization
    D. gender identify

4. What six criteria have been found useful for identifying the state of an individual's emotional health?

5. What are the four transitional periods in the life structure model proposed by Levinson and colleagues?

6. The term "human sexuality" does not refer to:
    A. health and well-being.
    B. sexual intercourse only.
    C. life-style.
    D. gender identity.

CHAPTER 11

Growth and Development Across the Life Span

■ **BEHAVIORAL OBJECTIVES**

After studying this chapter, you should be able to:

1. Describe attitudes of nurses that are helpful for assisting clients in all phases of growth and development.

2. Describe the essential nature of collaboration between the nurse and client as it relates to promoting human growth.

3. Define growth and development.

4. List five major principles of growth and development.

5. Describe the expected changes in physical growth and development across the life span.

6. Summarize major points about psychosocial development for each stage of the life span.

7. Describe the focus of nurse-client collaboration for promoting/maintaining normal growth and development of individuals at each stage of the life span.

8. List two common health problems for each stage of the life span.

9. Describe responsibilities of the nurse in collaborating with clients to manage common health problems encountered in each developmental phase of the life span.

■ **KEY TERMS**

accommodation
assimilation
attachment behaviors
cephalocaudal
cognitive development
critical periods
development
fine motor control

gross motor control
growth
individuation
learning disorder
magical thinking
maturation
moral development

object permanence
parallel play
phase
proximodistal
psychosocial development
puberty
therapeutic play

■ **REVIEW QUESTIONS**

1. List two behaviors or skills that nurses will find helpful for assisting clients in all phases of growth and development.

2. Define growth and development.

3. List five principles of growth and development.

4. Describe one expected change in physical growth and development for each of the following life stages.

    neonate

    infant

    toddler

    preschooler

school-age child

adolescent

young adult

middle-aged adult

older adult

5. Provide one major point of psychosocial development for each of the following life stages.

neonate

infant

toddler

preschooler

school-age child

adolescent

young adult

middle-aged adult

older adult

6. List two common health problems for each of the following life stages.

neonate

infant

toddler

preschooler

school-age child

adolescent

young adult

middle-aged adult

older adult

7. Define maturation.

8. Name two standardized tests nurses can use to measure maturational changes in children.

9. Identify the strategies nurses can use to assist older adults with transitional adjustments.

10. When does an infant develop a greater awareness of self as separate from mother or father? What is this called?

■ ENRICHMENT ACTIVITIES

1. Talk with a number of people you know who are parents (your own parents, those of friends, friends who are parents). Ask them where they got their information, skills, and beliefs about parenting. Do they use an intuitive approach, perhaps modeling their patterns after those of their own parents? How many mention a conscious effort to employ or avoid certain parenting patterns they experienced in their childhood? Do they ask friends for advice? Do they read books on the subject of parenting? Go to classes? Consult authorities? Which ones? Have they received parenting information from nurses? In what settings might nurses be in a position to counsel parents on parenting?

2. Safety is a human need that is served by intact senses; diminished hearing or vision can interfere with safety, but the impact will vary with the person's age. How might a loss of hearing in a 2-year-old child differ from

the same loss in a 14-year-old in its effect on safety needs? What implications would this have for a nurse caring for either client?

3. Talk to a person who has just become a parent for the first time about his or her primary concerns in caring for the infant. Then talk to someone who has two or more children, including an infant and an older child or teenager. How do the concerns of these two parents differ? Do their concerns relate to the developmental stage of the child or to their own sense of confidence in handling problems? Compare the overall sense of confidence projected. Which parent registers more concern and need for support? List the factors that might cause an experienced parent to have anxieties about child care.

4. Imagine you are interacting with individuals who represent various developmental stages: a 9-month-old infant, a 3-year-old child, a 10-year-old child, a 14-year-old teenager, a 21-year-old adult, a 52-year-old adult, and an 83-year-old adult. How might you be able to tell whether they trusted you? List specific behaviors (for each level) that might indicate trust.

5. Make a list of your family members; your parents, grandparents, great-grandparents, even great great-grandparents. Identify any significant health problems your ancestors might have had and their causes of death. Are any patterns apparent? Any illnesses that might be passed on from generation to generation? Any illnesses that might have been prevented? Given today's levels of health education and health care, could your ancestors' illnesses be prevented or controlled? Do any of your ancestors' illnesses pose health risks for you and others in your family? What preventive measures are appropriate?

■ SELF-EXAMINATION QUESTIONS

1. Which of the following statements is/are accurate?
    A. Knowledge of growth and development assists nurses to identify potential health decisions at different ages.
    B. Nurses can use knowledge of growth and development to evaluate the potential for a client's participation in decision making.
    C. There are no limitations in using collaboration to promote growth and development.
    D. Nurses using the collaborative approach can expect parents to readily disclose their ideas about growth and development.

2. Therapeutic play can best be described as:

3. Growth is:
    A. a quantitative term that describes physical change.
    B. a qualitative term that describes changes in function.
    C. both A and B.
    D. neither A nor B.

4. True or false: Infants display proximodistal, neuromuscular growth and development when they move both arms and hands together before using their fingers to handle objects.

5. True or false: Critical periods in growth and development refer to a cycle of changes.

6. What accounts for individual variations in patterns of growth and development?

7. List major tasks accomplished during the transition between adolescence and young adulthood.

8. Identify five physical changes in middle-aged and older adults that may affect their safety and well-being.

CHAPTER 12

Becoming a Client

■ **BEHAVIORAL OBJECTIVES**

After studying this chapter, you should be able to:

1. Describe the holistic perspective of health.

2. Identify variables affecting personal definitions of health.

3. Identify variables to health-seeking behavior in illness.

4. Define "sick role."

5. List two rights and two obligations inherent to the sick role.

6. Discuss the implication of the Szasz-Hollander model for client care.

7. Describe the three stages of illness and state key client problems in each stage.

8. Outline stress-provoking features of the hospital experience.

9. Describe several psychological responses to the hospital stay.

10. Discuss the importance of social class, ethnicity, and other cultural variables for nurse-client collaboration.

■ **KEY TERMS**

acute illness	chronic illness	illness behavior
bias	denial	locus of control
body image	holism	primary socialization

regression   self-care   social support
role   sick role   socialization
secondary socialization   social network

■ REVIEW QUESTIONS

1. Define the "sick role."

2. List two rights and two obligations inherent to the sick role.

   Rights:

   Obligations:

3. What is the implication of the Szasz-Hollander model for client care?

4. Identify the three stages of illness and state one key client problem for each stage.

5. List six stress-provoking features of the hospital experience.

6. Name seven psychological responses to the hospital stay.

7. What importance do interpersonal relationships play in relation to health risk?

8. Define the holistic perspective of health.

9. Identify three variables affecting personal definitions of health.

10. List five variables to health-seeking behavior in illness, using Mechanic's health belief model.

■ ENRICHMENT ACTIVITIES

1. Think of the last time someone in your family (or one of your friends) was ill. What were their symptoms? How did their activities affect their daily responsibilities? Did the relative change his or her routine? In what way? What was the response of other members of the family to these changes? What symptoms caused absence from work or school? What action did your relative take to alleviate the symptoms? Was a health care professional consulted? Why or why not? Would you say that your relative operated from a clinical or more personal definition of health and illness in responding to the situation?

2. Analyze your relative or friend's illness situation in terms of Rosenstock's Health Belief Model. In your opinion, how susceptible to illness did your relative perceive himself or herself to be? How serious did he or she regard the symptoms to be (life threatening, potentially disabling, no consequence, etc.)? What were the benefits of taking action such as seeking health advice (less worry, feel better, etc.), and what were the barriers to taking action (too expensive, lost day at work, etc.)? What cues from the environment did your relative use to make his or her health decisions in the situation (media information, friend's advice, etc.)?

3. Think of the last time you saw a health care professional about a personal health problem. Describe the relationship that developed in the encounter in terms of the Szasz-Hollander model. Were you given an active role in planning for the resolution of the problem? Would you describe the relationship as a collaborative one? Why or why not?

4. Think of the last time you had a health examination. What were some of the things that the health care professional did or failed to do to support your privacy and dignity in the situation? List some approaches they might have taken to help you feel more comfortable. Are any of these applicable to the clients you care for?

■ **SELF-EXAMINATION QUESTIONS**

1.   List the four main variables of the Rosenstock Health Belief Model.

2.   Which of the following is *not* one of Mechanic's 10 variables in the response to illness?
     A. the extent to which symptoms disrupt the individual's family, work, or other social activities
     B. the individual's perception of the health professional's knowledge about the symptoms
     C. the degree to which other needs compete with the illness response
     D. the alternative interpretations of symptoms considered by the individual

3.   True or false: The two obligations of the sick role according to Parsons are to seek professional help in order to overcome the disease, and to articulate the desire to get well.

4.   Describe the characteristics of the collaborative provider-client interaction.

5.   Which of the following *best* defines locus of control?
     A. Clients can be absolved from responsibility for control.
     B. Control is discussed by all involved participants in a situation.
     C. An individual's perception of the degree of personal control in a situation.
     D. The legal definition of responsibility to control in a specific situation.

CHAPTER 13

The Nurse–Client Relationship

■ **BEHAVIORAL OBJECTIVES**

After studying this chapter, you should be able to:

1. Discuss the characteristics of the following types of relationships: human to nonhuman, human to ideology, human to deity, and human to human.

2. Compare and contrast the professional and nonprofessional interpersonal (social) relationship.

3. Describe the characteristics of an effective helper.

4. Identify the three phases of the helping relationship as defined by Gazda and associates.

5. Explain the following concepts: empathy, respect, warmth, concreteness, genuineness, self-disclosure, confrontation, immediacy, trust, autonomy, and mutuality.

6. Identify at least one task of each of the four phases of the helping relationship as defined by Sundeen and associates.

7. Describe how collaboration occurs in each phase of the nurse-client relationship.

■ **KEY TERMS**

action phase	facilitation phase	manipulation
autonomy	genuineness	mutuality
concreteness	helping relationship	nurse-client relationship
confrontation	immediacy	orientation phase
contract	interpersonal relationship	preinteraction phase
empathy	intrapersonal relationship	respect

self-disclosure

sympathy

termination phase

therapeutic use of self

transition phase

value clarification

warmth

working phase

■ **REVIEW QUESTIONS**

1. Describe the characteristics of an effective helper.

2. Describe the three phases of Gazda's helping relationship.

3. Provide a one-sentence definition for each of the following terms.

    empathy

    respect

    warmth

    concreteness

    genuineness

    self-disclosure

    confrontation

    immediacy

    trust

autonomy

mutuality

4. Name one tool for each of the four phases of Sundeen's helping relationship.

5. Read each of the following statements. If the statement is true, mark it true. If the statement is false, correct the statement.

    A. In a professional relationship the helper's behavior reflects a balance between spontaneity and purposeful, planned interventions.

    B. In a nonprofessional relationship, sympathetic feelings for the other will not preclude or prevent helpful action.

6. Name one characteristic of each of the following types of relationships.

    human to nonhuman

    human to ideology

    human to deity

    human to human

7. What is the single most important element needed to develop effective nurse-client relationships?

8. List four characteristics of the trusting individual.

9. What is the most important tool available to nurses in assisting clients to meet health needs?

10. Name several advantages of using collaboration in the nurse-client relationship.

■ ENRICHMENT ACTIVITIES

1. Imagine that you will be taking care of a client for the morning. The extent of your responsibilities will be to assist the client with morning care, to make the bed, and to assess the client's dietary habits. Role play establishing a contract with this client. How do you feel about contracting? Some people find it dehumanizing. Do you agree or disagree with this point of view? Why?

2. Think of several examples of relationships you have had in the past. Discuss your own methods of dealing with those that terminated.   Is there anything you wish you had done differently?

3. Think about the characteristics that are essential to a collaborative, helping relationship--trust, empathy, autonomy, mutuality, warmth, confrontation, immediacy, and concreteness. Can you think of examples of relationships you have had in which these concepts were present? How did you feel in those relationships? Were they helpful to you? Why? Now think of relationships in which these characteristics were absent. How did these relationships make you feel? Why? How do you feel about implementing characteristics such as confrontation and immediacy within a helping relationship? You might want to practice the implementation of these characteristics with a classmate.

4. Imagine that you are in the hospital for surgery and a nursing student has been assigned to care for you. How would you want to be treated? After surgery, you experience incisional pain. What could the nursing student do for you that would be both helpful and collaborative?

■ SELF-EXAMINATION QUESTIONS

1. Match the term in column A with the appropriate definition in column B.

A	B
_____ (1) empathy	a. capacity for self-direction
_____ (2) trust	b. a process of sharing
_____ (3) autonomy	c. understanding what another may feel
_____ (4) mutuality	d. the assured belief that another will be supportive in time of stress
_____ (5) warmth	e. speaking in specifics
_____ (6) confrontation	f. dealing with the "here and now" of a relationship
_____ (7) immediacy	g. demonstration of caring
_____ (8) concreteness	h. communication of perceived discrepancies in behavior

2. True or false: An interpersonal relationship describes knowledge of self.

3. True or false: Sympathy contains the element of objectivity.

4. True or false: A contract addresses the purpose of the helping relationship.

5. In which phase of the helping relationship is a contract established?
    A. preinteraction
    B. orientation
    C. working
    D. termination

6. Which of the following actions characterizes the working phase of a helping relationship?
    A. assessment begun
    B. goal setting
    C. reflection on accomplishments
    D. contract setting

7. In carrying through on commitments made to a client, the nurse is demonstrating which of the following traits?
    A. empathy
    B. caring
    C. mutuality
    D. trustworthiness

8. The following statements refer to either a professional or a nonprofessional relationship. Use the following key to indicate which: professional = P, nonprofessional = N.

    _____ (1) Each participant responds to the other with help.

    _____ (2) The relationship is goal-directed.

    _____ (3) There is an explicit contract between the participants.

    _____ (4) Frequency of meetings is not predetermined.

CHAPTER 14

Communication as a Collaborative Process

■ **BEHAVIORAL OBJECTIVES**

After studying this chapter, you should be able to:

1. Define communication.

2. Identify five components of the communication process.

3. Discuss three processes necessary for the sharing of information.

4. Describe three major modes of communication.

5. State five goals of communication in nursing.

6. Explain the role of listening in the process of communication.

7. Identify and explain at least four approaches that support and six approaches that hinder collaborative communication.

8. Demonstrate empathy, warmth, respect, genuineness, concreteness, confrontation, and immediacy in actual or simulated nurse-client relationships.

9. Discuss variations in communication techniques that can be used with special populations such as the elderly, children, and clients of different cultural backgrounds.

10. Identify two types of interviews and describe situations in which each type would be most appropriate and effective.

11. Describe at least five approaches or guidelines for effective interviewing.

12. Describe the relationship of communication to the collaborative process.

■ **KEY TERMS**

assertive communication	incongruent communication	open-ended question
attending behavior	intergroup communications	perception
body language	internal feedback	personal distance
communication	interpersonal communication	person-to-group communication
connotative meaning	interview	receiver
context	intimate distance	response time
denotative meaning	intrapersonal communication	sender
direct question	language	social distance
empowering response	message	transmission
evaluation	metacommunication	verbal communication
feedback	nonverbal communication	

■ **REVIEW QUESTIONS**

1. Provide one or more definitions of communication.

2. List five components of the communication process.

3. List three processes necessary for the sharing of information.

4. Identify five goals of communication in nursing.

5. Discuss the role of listening in the communication process.

6.   Describe four approaches that support and four approaches that hinder communication.

7.   Name two types of interview and give appropriate examples for each.

8.   List five approaches or guidelines for effective interviewing.

9.   Provide an example of a communication technique that can be used with each of the following special populations.

elderly

children

different primary language

10.   Describe three modes of communication.

■ ENRICHMENT ACTIVITIES

1. With a friend discuss personal relationships characterized by the use of communication techniques presented in the chapter. How do such relationships make you feel?   More than likely they produce feelings of self-worth and respect within you. Now contrast those relationships with others that leave you feeling insecure and inadequate. Can you identify which communication techniques produce the good feelings and which the bad? Practice using the "good" approaches with your friend. Practice sometimes feels strange, but it is the best way to internalize approaches that are most beneficial in relationships.

2. Review the information on nonverbal attending behaviors. During the next week focus on these behaviors in others when you are at home, in school, or at work. What nonverbal attending behaviors seem most effective? What nonverbal behaviors are most hindering to the communication process?

3. The next time you and a friend are considering a decision regarding a mutual activity, practice the techniques of reflection, clarification, and attentive listening to explore what it is that your friend really wants to do. Once you have ascertained that information, try collaborating with your friend to decide on something that would please you both. As you proceed with this process, be aware of what is happening between the two of you; how do you feel?

4. Watch a television "soap opera." Write down the examples that you observe of ineffective communication. What are the results of the communication? How could things have turned out differently in the television show if the actors and actresses had used the communication approaches presented in this chapter?

5. As you become more aware of your own communication, note what your strengths are. Are you a good listener, but perhaps have difficulty making empathic responses? Or do you find listening a challenge? Whatever you identify as your strengths and weaknesses, make a commitment to consciously work on improving the area of deficiency. Work on one area at a time and be patient with yourself. A commitment to improve communication abilities will pay off in rich rewards in all relationships.

■ SELF-EXAMINATION QUESTIONS

1. Match the term in column A with the appropriate definition in column B.

<u>A</u>

_____ (1) verbal level of communication

_____ (2) connotative meaning

_____ (3) metacommunication

_____ (4) nonverbal meaning

_____ (5) denotative meaning

<u>B</u>

a. comprises over 60 percent of all communication

b. relates to a physical object as it exists in the world

c. a personal meaning

d. refers to words

e. the meaning behind words

2.   The examples in column A below illustrate communication occurring at specific levels. Match these examples with the levels that are listed in column B. The choices in column B may be used more than once.

<u>A</u>   <u>B</u>

_____ (1)   nurse interviewing a new client   a.   interpersonal communication

_____ (2)   nurse teaching 25 people about   b.   group communication
              AIDS
                                                           c.   intergroup communication
_____ (3)   nurse   reflecting   on   personal
              feelings   d.   intrapersonal communication

_____ (4)   ANA lobbying Congress for nurse
              traineeships

_____ (5)   nurse   teaching   new   mothers
              postpartum exercises

_____ (6)   nurse examining personal values
              on abortion

_____ (7)   nurse comforting dying adult

3.   Place a T next to the correct statements and an F next to the incorrect statements below.

_____ (1)   Verbal communication is comprised of action, object, and sign language.

_____ (2)   Warmth can be communicated nonverbally.

_____ (3)   Incongruent messages occur when the verbal and nonverbal messages are saying different things.

_____ (4)   The context in which communication occurs is important to the overall meaning of the message being transmitted.

_____ (5)   Effective listening is accomplished when the listener is subjective rather than objective.

4.   Match the statements in column A with the appropriate concept in column B.

<u>A</u>   <u>B</u>

_____ (1)   If it's important to you, then I want to listen.

a.   confrontation

b.   immediacy

_____ (2)   You've tried some things but so far nothing has worked. Tell me exactly what you have done.

c.   warmth

d.   concreteness

_____ (3)   I know this diet is difficult to follow but every week we talk about ways to make it manageable, yet your weight is not coming down.

e.   genuineness

_____ (4)   When I told you that I would have to cancel our meeting for next week, you seemed angry. Could we discuss your feelings?

_____ (5)   Sometimes when you tell me how your children treat you, I get angry with them.

CHAPTER 15

Professional Decision Making and the Nursing Process

■ **BEHAVIORAL OBJECTIVES**

After studying this chapter, you should be able to:

1. Define professional decision making.

2. Describe the advantages of a systematic, deliberative process such as the nursing process.

3. Discuss the use of nonsystematic approaches to decision making.

4. Compare the formats of the four nursing process models.

5. Describe the phases and steps of the Berger-Williams model.

6. Describe inductive and deductive reasoning processes for data collection.

7. Identify data evaluation strategies for improving data analysis.

8. Identify the factors in the decision environment that influence the complexity and uncertainty of professional decision making.

9. Describe three decision analysis methods for enhancing decision making.

10. Describe the characteristics of the decision maker that influence decision making.

11. Discuss the collaborative role of clients in health care decisions.

■ **KEY TERMS**

assessment phase
data analysis
data collection
decision analysis methods
decision environment
deductive reasoning
evaluation
heuristics

hypothesis
implementation
inductive reasoning
management phase
maximizing strategy
nursing diagnosis
nursing process
optimizing strategy

planning
preventive care
professional decision making
rehabilitative care
restorative care
satisficing
supportive care

■ **REVIEW QUESTIONS**

1. Define professional decision making.

2. List the activities of a systematic, deliberative process such as the nursing process.

3. Name and give an example of three nonsystematic approaches to decision making.

4. Identify the two phases of the Berger-Williams model.

5. Name the six steps of the Berger-Williams model.

6. Describe the differences between inductive and deductive reasoning processes for data collection.

7. Explain why inductive reasoning is or is not superior to deductive reasoning.

8. Identify three data evaluation strategies for improving data analysis.

9. Briefly describe four decision analysis methods that enhance decision making.

10. Name six characteristics of the decision maker that influence decision making.

■ **ENRICHMENT ACTIVITIES**

1. Observe health care professionals from different disciplines as they are involved in client care decision making. Are all health team members involved in the process? Why or why not? Is the client involved? Why or why not? What information was collected to make the necessary decisions? What alternative implementation strategies were considered? Were the potential benefits and costs of the outcomes considered? Was an evaluation plan developed?

2. Think about an important decision you have had to make. What was the nature of the decision? Choosing a college? Deciding on a course of study? Accepting or quitting a job? What information did you use to make the decision? Did you make a deliberate attempt to expand the information you had? Who or what sources did you consult for information? For advice? How did you approach the decision? Did you make a list of pros and cons? Did you weigh the various considerations according to how important they were to your decision? How much importance did you give to your emotions in making the decision? Would you say you made the decision on a consciously rational basis or did you use your intuition? Did personal habit play a role? How about authority? Were some people more influential in making your decision than others? What input from others was helpful?

3. Using the description in the text and the example in Figure 15-2, design a decision tree for the above decision that incorporates three outcomes to be achieved and three strategies or alternatives for achieving them. Be

sure to rank the outcomes in order of their importance to you. Is the decision reached by using this tool the same as the one you actually made? If not, what accounts for the discrepancy?

■ SELF-EXAMINATION QUESTIONS

1. Decision making in an open system includes all the following characteristics *except:*
    A. bounded rationality.
    B. incomplete knowledge of relevant factors.
    C. certainty of outcomes.
    D. multiple alternative actions.

2. A nonsystematic method of decision making by nurses is characterized by:
    A. scientific values.
    B. deliberation.
    C. bounded rationality.
    D. trial-and-error.

3. The nursing process is:
    A. an organizing framework for client-nurse decision making.
    B. an assessment of the client's history and health problems.
    C. a nonsystematic decision-making method.
    D. a static mechanism for meeting client care needs.

4. Identifying client-centered outcomes and implementation strategies is part of:
    A. the data collection step.
    B. the data analysis step.
    C. the planning step.
    D. the evaluation process.

5. A client who is moderately obese and has recently been diagnosed with mild hypertension requires nursing interventions at which level of care?
    A. preventive care
    B. supportive care
    C. restorative care
    D. rehabilitative care

6. True or false: Evaluation is a process of correction and adjustment.

CHAPTER 16

Client History and Health Examination

■ **BEHAVIORAL OBJECTIVES**

After studying this chapter, you should be able to:

1. List the elements of the data base for health assessment.

2. Differentiate subjective from objective data.

3. Define the health history and health examination and state their purposes; define subjective and objective manifestations.

4. Outline the elements of the health history and describe their contents.

5. Identify interview techniques that are appropriate to each phase of the health history.

6. Describe the procedure for height, weight, and other body measurements.

7. Define body temperature, describe factors that regulate and alter it, outline the procedure for measuring oral, rectal, and axillary temperatures, and discuss the expected findings.

8. Define respiration, describe factors that regulate and alter it, outline the procedure for measuring respiration, and discuss the expected findings.

9. Define pulse, describe factors that regulate and alter it, outline the procedure for measuring apical and peripheral pulses, and discuss the expected findings.

10. Define blood pressure, describe factors that regulate and alter it, outline the procedure for measuring blood pressure by auscultation, palpation, and flush methods, and discuss the expected findings.

11. Outline the order of the head-to-toe examination.

12. Define inspection, palpation, percussion, and auscultation.

13. List several observations for each body area and system included in the health examination and identify the method of observation appropriate for each.

14. Relate observations of the head-to-toe examination to the nurse's role.

15. State the purpose of health assessment by nurses and describe the nurse's focus in doing a health assessment.

16. Discuss the importance of collaboration in the health history and examination.

■ KEY TERMS

auscultation	Korotkoff sounds	pulse rhythm
basal metabolic rate	medical data base	pulse symmetry
blood pressure	nursing data base	pulse volume
body temperature	objective data	radiation
chest vibration	ophthalmoscope	respiration
conduction	otoscope	respiratory depth
convection	palpation	respiratory rate
data base	percussion	respiratory rhythm
diastolic blood pressure	point of maximal impulse	respiratory quality
evaporation	precordium	sphygmomanometer
health assessment	pulse	subjective data
health examination	pulse pressure	systolic blood pressure
health history	pulse rate	turgor
inspection		

■ REVIEW QUESTIONS

Mr. R, a 72-year-old man, has just been wheeled into the health center emergency room after suffering a "black-out spell." He was brought in by the ambulance driver. His daughter plans to come to the health center as soon as she finds someone to watch her 4-year-old child. A nurse in the hallway says "I'll be right back" as Mr. R. is wheeled by her. Ten minutes later Mr. R. is still sitting alone in his wheelchair in the examining room.

1. What would you have done differently in this situation?

2. List five things that could have been done to make this a more comfortable experience for Mr. R.

As Mr. R. is being helped into an examining gown he says, "I don't remember what happened. I was getting up from the kitchen chair, and the next thing I knew I was on the floor! My left hand feels sort of tingly."

3. List three examples of **subjective** data the nurse can gather from this encounter.

4. List three types of **objective** data a nurse might gather from clinical observation of Mr. R.

5. Give an example of two kinds of questions that might be used in a nursing assessment and interview with this client.

6. After you have finished the questions for your planned interview, what questions could you ask to obtain additional unplanned information?

7. What is the purpose of inspection and palpation?

8. Describe the difference between direct and indirect percussion.

9. What is the purpose and technique of using the (A) bell and (B) diaphragm portions of the stethoscope?

10. Give an example of three questions you could ask to assess Mr. R.'s neurologic status.

11. Name eight body measurements a nurse might make in conducting a health examination.

12. What are some of the factors that influence body temperature?

13. What are some of the factors that influence respiration?

14. Name four characteristics of a pulse.

15. Distinguish between systolic and diastolic blood pressure.

16. Define general assessment and list at least five observations nurses make as part of the inspection stage of a general head-to-toe assessment.

17. Identify four techniques that are commonly used in a general assessment.

18. For the following body systems, provide the following assessment information: (1) two client history questions for subjective manifestations of illness; (2) four objective manifestation findings; and (3) one special consideration, precaution, or source of error that may arise during assessment. Enter your answers on a separate sheet of paper.

    Systems: integument; head, face, and nose; ear; eye; mouth and throat; neck; breasts and axillae; thorax and lungs; cardiovascular system; abdomen and gastrointestinal system; anus and rectum; genitourinary system; musculoskeletal system; neurological system

■ ENRICHMENT ACTIVITIES

1. Recall your last personal medical office visit. Write down both your physical and psychological responses to what occurred while you were seated in the waiting room. How did the office personnel help or fail to help you feel comfortable? Which of these approaches would benefit your clients?

2. Compile a list of the body systems evaluated during the health examination and list the equipment used when examining each system.

3. Practice listening to the percussion sound differences that occur when percussing a puffed-out cheek, the thigh muscle, and the ankle bone. You might even try "percussing" the walls of your room. Can you locate the vertical beams that constitute the frame of the wall? What sounds helped you locate them? How did these sounds compare with the sounds created by percussing your ankle bone?

4. Think of the last health examination you had. What did the examiner do to include you in the examination process? Would you describe your relationship with the examiner as collaborative? Why or why not?

5. Take your pulse while at rest. Observe its rate and quality. Then exercise for a few minutes. Again observe your pulse rate and quality. What differences did you observe? Name the nervous reflexes that participate in pulse changes.

■ **SELF-EXAMINATION QUESTIONS**

1. Identify the exact placement of a correctly applied blood pressure cuff.

2. Convert a Fahrenheit temperature of 100.0° to centigrade.

3. When weighing a client, which of the following procedures apply?
    A. Have the client void before being weighed.
    B. Weigh the client at the same time each day before breakfast.
    C. Have the client wear the same clothing each time he or she is weighed.
    D. All of the above procedures should be followed.

4. How is taking an apical-radial pulse different from taking other pulse measurements?

5. List the components of the health history that are elicited by the nurse.

CHAPTER 17

Nursing Diagnosis

■ **BEHAVIORAL OBJECTIVES**

After studying this chapter, you should be able to:

1. Define nursing diagnosis and differentiate it from medical diagnosis.

2. Identify the relationship of nursing diagnosis to nursing process.

3. Trace the historical development of nursing diagnosis.

4. Define taxonomy.

5. Summarize the progress to date and future directions in the development of nursing's diagnostic taxonomy.

6. Identify the components of a nursing diagnosis statement.

7. Formulate nursing diagnosis statements from the list of approved diagnoses, their etiologies, and defining characteristics.

8. Differentiate the methods of stating actual and potential nursing diagnoses.

9. Outline the process of diagnostic reasoning.

10. Describe the most common type of diagnostic error and its sources.

11. Correlate several common sources of diagnostic error with the novice and the expert.

12. Identify six advantages of nursing diagnosis to nursing practice.

■ KEY TERMS

category label

contributing factor

cue

defining characteristic

diagnostic label

diagnostic reasoning

etiology

inference

inferential leap

manifestation

nursing diagnosis

organizational framework

PES format

potential diagnosis

problem

related factor

risk factor

taxonomy

■ REVIEW QUESTIONS

1. Explain the differences between a nursing diagnosis and a medical diagnosis.

2. What is the relationship of nursing diagnosis to the nursing process?

3. Name an outcome of the initial conference on nursing diagnosis held in 1973.

4. Define taxonomy.

5. Identify the three components of a nursing diagnosis statement.

6. Formulate nursing diagnosis statements for the following four approved diagnoses, their etiologies, and their defining characteristics.

   pain

   constipation

   activity intolerance

   self-esteem disturbance

7. Explain the difference between stating actual and potential nursing diagnoses.

8. Distinguish between a cue and an influence.

9. Describe the most common type of diagnostic error and its sources.

10. Identify six advantages of nursing diagnosis for nursing practice.

■ ENRICHMENT ACTIVITIES

For each of the following cases, formulate appropriate nursing diagnoses. Work individually or in small groups. Compare your diagnoses with those of classmates and discuss differences, if any. Compare your answers with the answer key. If your diagnoses differ, try to identify your errors in diagnostic reasoning.

Case Study 1:

Jessica Jones, a 63-year-old school teacher, has been admitted to the medical ward with the medical diagnosis: Type II diabetes mellitus (DM). The diagnosis is the outcome of a preretirement physical examination. Mrs. Jones is obese: ht 5'4", wt 200 lbs; her fasting blood sugar (FBS) is 400.

Mrs. Jones has recently been widowed, her husband succumbed to a "stroke" 6 months ago. She has no children, and her only sibling lives in a distant state.

Upon entering Mrs. Jones' room, the nurse finds her weeping into her pillow. When questioned about her behavior, Mrs. Jones sobs, "I'm so scared. My mother died from diabetes. Her diet was terrible and she had to take those awful shots. The one joy I have left in life is eating and now that's being taken way."

Case Study 2:

Sally Strong, a 52-year-old telephone operator, is 6 hours postcholecystectomy. Over the past 4 hours you have gathered the following assessment data:
- Pinched brow; facial mask of discomfort.
- Reluctance to move, reposition in bed.
- Refusal to participate in deep breathing, coughing exercises; states, "I'll start tomorrow, I promise."
- Full participation in active leg exercises.
- Demonstrated sound understanding of principles underlying postoperative rehabilitative regime.
- 2 packs per day smoker x 30 years.
- Ht 5'5", wt 164 lbs.
- HR 70, reg; RR 24, shallow and asymmetrical; BP 100/72; afebrile.
- Lung auscultation: crackles R base, diminished breath sounds both bases.
- No BM x 2 days.
- Bowel sounds absent x 4 quadrants.
- NG tube to low/intermittent suction, draining thin, light-green material.

■ **SELF-EXAMINATION QUESTIONS**

1.   Give at least three definitions of nursing diagnosis.

2.   Nursing diagnosis:
     A. helps ensure a discipline-specific perspective for professional nurses.
     B. can be summarized in a single, concise definition.
     C. forms the basis for interventions by other disciplines.
     D. is a subjective assessment.

3.   True or false: Use of the term "inference" in nursing diagnosis emphasizes the tentative and assumptive nature of the process.

4.   True or false: A frequent source of diagnostic error for the novice nurse is the tendency to prematurely terminate the analysis of cues.

5.   What are the components of the PES format?

6.   For each of the following problem statements: (1) evaluate whether the criteria for stating a nursing diagnosis are met; (2) if not, specify why, and how the statement might be modified to meet the criteria. Note that each problem statement is accompanied by either an etiology or risk factors, yet defining characteristics accompany none of the problem statements, purposefully.

     A. Chronic Bronchitis R/T hypertrophy of pulmonary mucus glands.
     B. Anorexia R/T side effects of chemotherapy.
     C. Abdominal Distention R/T malfunctioning nasogastric tube suction apparatus.
     D. Knowledge Deficit: low sodium diet R/T lack of previous exposure to dietary restriction, and need for same.

E. Altered Nutrition: Potential for More Than Body Potassium Requirements, Risk Factors: potassium-sparing diuretic therapy, and use of salt substitutes.
F. Impaired Home Maintenance Management R/T decreased cardiac output.
G. Social Isolation R/T body image disturbance.
H. Fear R/T misconceptions regarding surgery.

CHAPTER 18

Making, Writing, and Evaluating Client Care Plans

■ **BEHAVIORAL OBJECTIVES**

After studying this chapter, you should be able to:

1. Define the terms desired outcome, nursing implementation, evaluation criteria, and evaluation.

2. List the benefits of the individualized client care plan.

3. Identify criteria for priority setting.

4. List elements to be considered when establishing deadlines for desired outcomes.

5. Formulate desired outcome statements that are specific, client oriented, and measurable.

6. State the major differences between long-term and short-term outcomes.

7. Describe the proper format for a nursing implementation statement.

8. Describe possible differences and similarities between evaluation criteria and desired outcome statements.

9. Describe four activities involved in the evaluation phase of the nursing process.

10. State the difference between situational and structured reporting.

11. Identify the characteristics of effective reporting.

12. State guidelines for recording information on the client's chart.

13. State the benefits of collaborative planning for the client and the nurse.

14. Identify two types of evaluation used to determine the quality of client care.

15.   Describe the purpose and steps of a quality assurance evaluation.

■ **KEY TERMS**

audit   formative evaluation   problem-oriented record
client care plan   independent functions   quality assurance program
client record   interdependent functions   retrospective evaluation
collaborative functions   Kardex   short-term outcome
dependent functions   long-term outcome   source-oriented record
desired outcome   monitoring   standard care plan
discharge planning   nursing implementation   standard of care
evaluation   nursing order   summative evaluation
evaluation criterion   priority setting

■ **REVIEW QUESTIONS**

1.   Define the following terms:

     desired outcome statement

     nursing implementation

     evaluation criteria

2.   List six benefits of the individualized collaborative client care plan.

3.   Briefly describe four priorities for developing a client care plan.

4. List three elements to consider when establishing deadlines for desired outcomes.

5. Identify four guidelines for writing outcome statements that are specific, client-oriented and measurable.

6. State the major differences between long-term and short-term outcomes.

7. Describe the four activities involved in evaluating client care plans.

8. Identify the five characteristics of effective reporting.

9. Briefly describe two types of evaluation used to determine the quality of client care plans.

10. Describe the purpose and steps of a quality assurance program.

■ ENRICHMENT ACTIVITIES

1. The next time you are in the clinical area, ask a nurse for samples of several types of flowsheets used in that unit. Bring the flowsheets home and practice filling in the data requested on each sheet. What types of data are recorded on each kind of flowsheet? Are all flowsheets used for every client? What determines whether a client has a flowsheet in his or her chart?

2. Watch an episode of your favorite TV drama. Pick one of the characters and imagine the character being admitted to the hospital for diagnostic tests for abdominal pain. Based on what you know of the character, write a care plan that anticipates the client care problems that might occur while the individual is hospitalized. Consider doing this exercise with a fellow student. After writing your care plans, compare them. Did you identify similar potential problems for the character?

3. Imagine that a family member is hospitalized for an undiagnosed illness that involves pain in one leg and difficulty ambulating. Based on what you know about your relative, write an individualized client care plan that anticipates the nursing problems your relative would be likely to have.

4. Ask a few of your close friends or relatives about their experiences in the hospital. Were they aware of a "plan" for their care? Ask what the nurses did on their behalf and whether these activities related to their primary concerns. Why is it important to know the client's primary concern? What is the importance of the primary concern in formulating an individualized care plan?

■ SELF-EXAMINATION QUESTIONS

1. List four activities involved in the planning phase of the nursing process.

2. Factor(s) that influence the setting of priorities include(s):
    A. the client's cultural beliefs and practices.
    B. the amount of assistance the client needs.
    C. the urgency of the problem.
    D. B and C.
    E. all of the above.

3. Differentiate between formative, summative, and retrospective evaluation. Include the purpose of each.

4. In order to formulate clear and succinct desired outcome statements, a nurse should do what five things?

5. Institutional evaluation of the quality of client care:
    A. occurs through the quality assurance program.
    B. grew out of legislation enacted to monitor cost and quality of care.
    C. focuses on structure, process, and outcome.
    D. all of the above.

6. List four components that each nursing implementation statement *must* have.

CHAPTER 19

Collaborating with the Health Care Team

■ **BEHAVIORAL OBJECTIVES**

After studying this chapter, you should be able to:

1. Describe the components of a team.

2. Describe the three stages of group development and outline several principles of group dynamics.

3. Outline the role and complementary functions of members of the health care team.

4. Discuss the need for collaboration among health care professionals.

5. Identify the aims of collaboration within the health care team.

6. Describe the complementary nature of medical and nursing diagnoses.

7. Discuss two factors that determine the nature of a collaborative professional relationship.

8. List modes of collaboration seen in health care settings.

9. Compare the roles of the initiator and maintainer in relation to group dynamics.

10. Explain how nurses can take on the role of initiator and maintainer in the health care team.

11. List four behaviors that nurses can use to facilitate collaboration of team members and participation of clients in the decision-making process.

12. Describe the importance of clients' participation as a member of the health care team.

13. Identify potential obstacles to collaboration among health care team members.

14. Discuss intrinsic and extrinsic factors that facilitate collaboration among team members.

15. Describe potential ethical issues related to collaboration.

■ **KEY TERMS**

accountability   collaboration   health care team conference
advocacy   consolidated client record   laissez-faire
assertiveness   consultation   risk taking
authoritarian   democratic   team
autocratic   detente   territoriality
autonomy   group dynamics
cohesiveness

■ **REVIEW QUESTIONS**

1. List the six characteristics of a team.

2. Identify the three stages of group development.

3. Describe the primary role of the health care team and the collaborative functions of the team members.

4. Name two factors that describe the nature of a collaborative professional relationship.

5. Describe the roles of the initiator and the maintainer in relation to group dynamics.

6. Provide examples of how nurses can take on the roles of initiator and maintainer in the health care team.

7. List four behaviors that nurses can use to foster collaboration among team members and participation of clients in the decision-making process.

8. Identify potential obstacles to collaboration among health care team members.

9. List the intrinsic and extrinsic factors that facilitate collaboration among health care members.

10. Describe two potential ethical issues related to collaboration.

■ ENRICHMENT ACTIVITIES

1. Communication is an integral aspect of collaboration. Several different styles of communication may be apparent within the health care team. Mechanisms that foster the development of collaborative relationships may be identified by analyzing communication patterns.

    Respond to the following questions. Consider aspects of your own communication style in different situations. Refer to the following sections for further information: Communication as a Collaborative Practice, Chapter 14; The Nature of a Collaborative Relationship, Chapter 19.

    A. Would you describe your overall communication style as "open" or "closed"? Justify your response.

    B. How do you communicate in a group versus communicating with one or two individuals?

    C. Do you assume that everyone understands what you are communicating or do you attempt to elicit feedback from others regarding their understanding?

    D. Do you use listening as part of your communication style? Give some examples of how listening may be incorporated into communication.

    E. Compare and contrast how you communicate verbally and nonverbally.

2. You have just completed your assessment of a client. You read the physician's assessment and find information in it that contradicts your own assessment. Discuss the steps you might take to communicate and share information about the discrepancies. Use the following questions to guide your response.

    A. Would you approach the client or physician first about these discrepancies? Why?

    B. Would you assume that the physician's information is more accurate? Why or why not?

    C. Would you document your information in the client care record without collaborating with the health care team? Why or why not?

    D. What would be some consequences if collaboration among health care team members did not occur in such a situation?

    E. How does your professional accountability relate to such a situation?

3. The term group dynamics refers to the processes or activities a group performs as part of its interactions. Consider your pattern of interactions in a group to which you belong. It may be your clinical group or another formal group. Draw a diagram that maps the patterns of interactions among group members. Examine the diagram and respond to the following questions.

    A. Which group members lead the discussion?

    B. Which group members communicate more frequently with one another?

    C. Which group members tend to be listeners?

    D. Does there seem to be more one-way or more two-way communication among group members?

E. Are there group members who do not communicate with each other?

F. Would you describe the overall pattern of communication as collaborative? Why or why not?

4. Norms are rules developed by a group to encourage conformity in the actions and attitudes of its members. As a new nursing student, you have had to learn some new norms. Consider both the school and hospital setting. Respond to the following questions:

A. What explicit norms have you encountered in your new role as a nursing student?

B. What implicit norms have you encountered? How were these norms brought to your attention?

5. Watch a television show or film that deals with health care. Examine how the media portray the working relationships among health care team members. Answer the following questions:

A. How would you categorize the working relationships among the health care team members (i.e., authoritarian, detente, collaborative)?

B. Can you identify obstacles to the development of collaboration as portrayed in the show?

C. If collaboration does occur, what factors enhance collaboration?

D. How do you think the public would respond to the relationships among health care professionals as portrayed in the show?

■ SELF-EXAMINATION QUESTIONS

1.   The nature of a collaborative relationship is determined by:
     A. professional exchange and mutual respect.
     B. the policies of the health care institution.
     C. the degree of specialization of the health care professionals.
     D. assertiveness and risk taking by team members.

2.   In the first stage of team growth, the orientation phase, tasks of the group members usually include:
     A. identifying norms and planning teamwork.
     B. developing cohesion and a common group language.
     C. learning expectations and developing trust in others.
     D. determining who is in control and developing a "we" identity.

3.   In comparing medical to nursing diagnoses, the focus of medicine is on _____, whereas the focus of nursing is on _____.

4.   The role of initiator in a group includes all of the following tasks *except.*
     A. synthesizing information to pull ideas together.
     B. introducing or proposing objectives to meet client needs.
     C. focusing the group on a particular task.
     D. harmonizing team members to minimize differences.

5. A head nurse who includes nursing staff in the decision-making processes regarding plans to implement a computerized care planning system is using:
    A. decision-centered leadership.
    B. laissez-faire leadership.
    C. democratic leadership.
    D. authoritarian leadership.

6. Which of the following terms refers to taking responsibility for one's actions and behaviors?
    A. accountability
    B. assertiveness
    C. risk taking
    D. aggressiveness

CHAPTER 20

Teaching and Learning as Collaboration

■ **BEHAVIORAL OBJECTIVES**

After studying this chapter, you should be able to:

1. Define teaching and learning.

2. Describe how each of the steps in the teaching-learning process is carried out collaboratively.

3. Discuss social and professional factors that support client teaching as an integral aspect of client health care.

4. Compare and contrast the definitions of learning and the premises about how learning occurs in behaviorism and the Gestalt-field theory.

5. Describe the types of behaviors that are characteristic of each of the three domains of learning.

6. Discuss the mental operations that are necessary to acquire and process information.

7. List and discuss factors that contribute to an individual's readiness, ability, and learning style.

8. Identify components of the standard health assessment that produce data relevant to health teaching.

9. Identify elements of a client's support system that may influence learning and/or application of health-related knowledge in daily activities. Discuss how these elements may be assessed and incorporated in the teaching-learning process.

10. Discuss at least four etiologies of the Knowledge Deficit nursing diagnosis, explaining how each contributes to a knowledge deficit.

11. Name and describe the components of a teaching-learning plan and form behavioral objectives for such a plan.

12. Compare and contrast informal and structured health teaching and describe situations in which each is appropriate.

13. Discuss the advantages and disadvantages of individual and group teaching approaches and describe situations in which each would be more appropriate.

14. Describe teaching approaches and teaching aids that are appropriate for health teaching.

15. Describe three ways in which client learning may be validated.

■ **KEY TERMS**

behavior	knowledge deficit	prompt
behavioral objective	learning	readiness
cognitive style	learning domain	response
conditioned response	learning objective	return demonstration
conditioned stimulus	literacy	secondary reinforcement
conditioning	negative reinforcement	simultaneous mutual interaction
feedback	positive reinforcement	stimulus
field	primary reinforcement	teaching
Gestalt	prime	

■ **REVIEW QUESTIONS**

1. Provide brief definitions for teaching and learning.

2. Name four social factors that support client teaching as an integral part of health care for clients.

3. List three professional factors that support client teaching as an integral part of health care for clients.

4. Match the theorists in column A with the correct theories in column B.

<u>A</u>

_____ (1) Bandura

_____ (2) Rogers

_____ (3) Bloom

_____ (4) Simpson

<u>B</u>

a. described three domains of learning.

b. developed a model of seven levels of psychomotor learning

c. contends that imitation or modeling is the basis of learning

d. the need to attain a feeling of personal adequacy is seen as a major factor that drives learning

5. Estimates indicate that approximately 27 million adults in the United States are functionally illiterate. What does the term "functionally illiterate" mean?

6. Name three of the six possible etiologies for the Knowledge Deficit diagnosis.

7. List four factors that can influence a client's readiness for health teaching.

8. Identify the three major characteristics of learners that can influence learning.

9. Match the teaching methods in column A with the correct descriptions in column B.

A

_____ (1) lecture

_____ (2) discussion

_____ (3) role-playing

_____ (4) behavior-rehearsal

_____ (5) demonstration-coaching

_____ (6) teaching aids

B

a. AVs, pictures, and diagrams that enhance a presentation

b. sequential steps or levels that help learners achieve progressively higher levels of proficiency

c. learners play themselves in imagined situations

d. involves acting out a real-life situation and follow-up discussion

e. verbal exchange of ideas between two or more persons

f. one-way transmission of verbal messages from teacher to learner

10. Identify three considerations important to implementation of a teaching-learning plan.

■ ENRICHMENT ACTIVITIES

1. Recall learning experiences you have had that stand out in your mind--experiences such as learning to drive, to ride a bicycle, to solve a math problem. Evaluate those experiences according to whether you feel the teaching you received was successful or unsuccessful. List characteristics of the teachers involved and the teaching strategies they used that were effective and ineffective. What positive approaches did you experience that you might want to carry over into your role of teaching clients?

2. Think about yourself as the learner in those experiences. What learning theory best describes how you mastered the tasks or concepts involved? Behaviorism? Gestalt-field? Social learning? Share descriptions of past learning experiences with a classmate. Together, analyze the techniques and strategies used by your teachers in terms of the learning theory they best represent. Discuss your rationale.

3. Pick up a copy of a magazine, booklet, or pamphlet used to educate consumers about health. Examine the material for content, readability, use of illustrations, photos, and graphics. Is the material useful? Engaging? Are the topics relevant to consumer needs and interests? Are enough facts presented? Too many? Are the illustrations helpful?

4. Imagine that a relative you know particularly well is told that he or she needs surgery for a condition that is not life-threatening. Write a teaching plan for your relative to prepare him or her for the surgery. What

factors about your relative do you feel are especially important to consider in writing the plan? Is age a factor? What about education level? Will terminology or vocabulary be a factor? Is there a language barrier to deal with? Is your relative's vision or hearing a potential barrier? Has your relative had prior experiences with surgery or being in a hospital? Does this need to be considered?

■ **SELF-EXAMINATION QUESTIONS**

1. You are teaching a group of hypersensitive clients about high blood pressure and about the possibilities for controlling it by modifying life-style. You stress the need to reduce cardiac risk factors, get regular exercise, and eat a low-salt, low-fat diet. Match the client statements in column A with the appropriate type of learning in column B. (NOTE: The same answer may be used more than once in column A.)

<u>A</u>   <u>B</u>

_____ (1) "I don't feel that I have a problem   a. psychomotor
              because I don't take any medicine."
                                                                                        b. cognitive
_____ (2) "My favorite food for lunch is a
              McDonald's hamburger and french   c. affective
              fries."
                                                                                        d. affective/cognitive
_____ (3) "The doctor says my blood pressure
              is 220/110. What should it be?"

_____ (4) "When I listen through the ear
              plugs, and let air out of the cuff, I
              don't hear any sounds at all!"

_____ (5) "I just love popcorn. Can I eat
              popcorn made without salt?"

2. A client is performing a return demonstration of a procedure he needs to master. During the demonstration the nurse can promote learning by:
    A. telling the client his performance is about as expected.
    B. counseling the client about the consequences of his errors.
    C. exhorting the client to do better.
    D. praising the client when his performance is accurate.

CHAPTER 21

Computers as an Aid to Collaboration

■ **BEHAVIORAL OBJECTIVES**

After studying this chapter, you should be able to:

1. Differentiate between computer hardware and computer software and describe the function of the various parts of the computer.

2. Describe five applications of computers in clinical practice.

3. Identify four advantages of computer use by nurses in clinical practice.

4. Identify three disadvantages of computer use by nurses in clinical practice.

5. Discuss the issues of privacy, confidentiality, and security as they relate to computer use by nurses.

6. Describe four types of computer-assisted instruction.

7. Discuss how computer-assisted instruction can be used in nursing education.

8. Discuss how computer-assisted instruction can be used in client education.

9. List three ways computers can assist nurses in conducting research.

10. List four computer applications used by nursing administrators.

11. Describe three types of general applications software.

12. Discuss how computers aid in collaboration among health care professionals in nursing practice, nursing education, nursing research, and nursing administration.

■ KEY TERMS

arithmetic/logical unit
assembly language
bit
byte
central processing unit
computer
computer-assisted instruction

control unit
hardware
high-level language
hospital information systems
machine language
microchip
microprocessor

primary memory
programs
random-access memory
read-only memory
secondary memory
software

■ REVIEW QUESTIONS

1. Name five applications of computers in clinical practice.

2. Identify four advantages of computer use by nurses in clinical practice.

3. List three disadvantages of computer use by nurses in clinical practice.

4. Match the terms in column A with the appropriate descriptions in column B.

<u>A</u>

_____ (1) drill and practice

_____ (2) tutorial programs

_____ (3) simulations

_____ (4) interactive video

<u>B</u>

a. combines computer-assisted instruction (CAI) with a videodisc

b. real-life situations are presented to learners, allowing interaction-development of problem-solving and decision-making skills in a safe environment

c. presents information, asks a learner to answer questions about it, and provides feedback

d. presents the learner with a series of questions or problems about already-learned material and allows the learner to master a topic through repeated practice; well suited for drug calculations

5. List three ways computers can assist nurses in conducting research.

6. Name four computer applications used by nursing administrators.

7. Describe three types of general computer applications software.

8. Name two decision support systems.

9. List two resources nurses can use to identify new software.

10. Describe three data bases that are helpful to nurses conducting literature searches.

■ ENRICHMENT ACTIVITIES

1. Visit the computer center in your school. What types of computer hardware are available? Identify the general-purpose software and nursing software available. If you are unfamiliar with either the equipment or software, inquire about orientation assistance available at the center.

2. Visit a store that sells computers and computer software. Before the visit, identify what you and your family might use a computer for; for example, preparing papers for school, playing games, keeping track of home finances. Talk with the salesperson about which computer would be best for your needs. Identify the type of hardware, disk drives, monitor, and amount of memory recommended as well as the cost of the various recommendations. Ask about software packages to meet your projected computer needs. What do the software packages cost, and can they be run on the recommended hardware?

3. Review a computer-assisted instruction (CAI) program. Identify the type of CAI program. Was the program clearly presented and well organized? Was the content accurate? What type of feedback did the program provide the learner? Was it individualized? How were incorrect answers and typographical errors handled? Were there programmed "help" messages to assist you in running the program? What were the strengths and weaknesses of the program? Identify potential uses of the program.

4. Do a tutorial-type CAI program. Describe how a tutorial-type computer program could be used for client education.

5. Visit a local hospital where the staff nurses use a computer and talk with nurses about what they use the computer for, how they learned to use the computer, and what they see as the advantages and disadvantages of the computer.

■ SELF-EXAMINATION QUESTIONS

1. The IBM-PC and the Apple computers are examples of what type of computer?
    A. mainframe computer
    B. minicomputer
    C. microcomputer
    D. all of the above

2. Which of the following has *not* been shown to be an advantage of hospital information systems?
    A. error reduction
    B. time saving
    C. protection of client privacy
    D. legibility of computer output

3. Most CAI software today runs on what type of computer?
    A. mainframe computer
    B. minicomputer
    C. microcomputer
    D. all of the above

4. All of the following are required to communicate with someone via computer *except*:
    A. a phone line.
    B. a modem.
    C. telecommunications software.
    D. a floppy disk.

5. The MEDLINE database includes citations found in all of the following indexes *except*:
    A. *International Nursing Index.*
    B. *Cumulative Index to Nursing and Allied Health Literature.*
    C. *Index Medicus.*
    D. *Index to Dental Literature.*

6. Which type of general-purpose computer software would be most useful to the nursing administrator in planning a budget?
    A. word processor
    B. database manager
    C. spreadsheet
    D. telecommunications

7. An administrative computer system that assigns nursing staff daily based on client acuity is called a:
    A. patient classification system.
    B. unit staffing system.
    C. scheduling system.
    D. quality assurance system.

CHAPTER **22**

Wellness and Well-being

■ **BEHAVIORAL OBJECTIVES**

After studying this chapter, you should be able to:

1. Define the concepts of health, wellness, and well-being.

2. Discuss the development of the wellness movement in the United States.

3. Discuss the relationship between the health of the individual and life-style practices.

4. Describe the basic elements of a wellness life-style.

5. Describe the objective and subjective manifestations of wellness and altered wellness.

6. Identify several factors that enhance or alter wellness.

7. Identify the wellness tasks related to various developmental stages.

8. Describe the impact of illness on wellness.

9. Discuss elements of health care experiences that can influence an individual's level of wellness.

10. Outline the elements of the health history that are pertinent to assessing wellness and well-being.

11. Discuss the implications of selected objective manifestations for assessing wellness and well-being.

12. Discuss the role of diagnostic tests in assessing wellness.

13. List the nursing diagnoses that are most commonly associated with altered wellness and well-being.

14. Describe preventive care measures for wellness and well-being.

15. State the relevance of self-management techniques for making life-style changes.

16. Describe supportive, restorative, and rehabilitative care measures available to assist clients with altered wellness or well-being.

17. List the nurse's responsibilities for admission of the client to the hospital.

18. Define medical and surgical asepsis and describe nursing procedures aimed at preventing nosocomial infection.

19. Discuss ways nurses can support and enhance the wellness and well-being of clients who are receiving treatment for health alterations.

20. Discuss the nurse's role in assisting the client with stress and describe several stress management techniques.

21. Discuss the nurse's role in reducing environmental hazards and reducing accidents.

22. Outline the nurse's role in managing fever.

23. Outline the principles of safe medication administration.

24. Describe the procedures for giving medication by the oral, subcutaneous, intramuscular, intravenous, rectal, and vaginal routes.

25. Describe the procedures for eye and ear instillations.

26. Describe three systems of measurement in current use for prescribing drugs.

27. State the formula for medication dosage calculation.

28. Outline the key aspects of the care of the client prior to, during, and after surgery.

■ **KEY TERMS**

absorption	locus of control	self-efficacy
ampule	medical asepsis	side effect
anaphylaxis	medication	stat order
chemical name	metabolism	sterile technique
distribution	nosocomial infection	subcutaneous
drug	official name	surgical asepsis
drug tolerance	patient-controlled analgesia	therapeutic effect
excretion	perioperative nursing	toxic effect
fitness	potentiation	trade name
generic name	privacy	universal precautions
hardiness	prn order	vial
intradermal	proprietary name	well-being
intramuscular	relaxation response	wellness
intravenous	resilience	

■ **REVIEW QUESTIONS**

1. Give a brief overview of the wellness movement.

2. Discuss how nursing fits into the history of the wellness model.

3. Mary Morrisey is a 59-year-old married woman with two adult children. She was diagnosed as having non-insulin dependent diabetes about three years ago. When you visit with her you focus on how well she is and how able she is to care for herself. What would you look for to determine how well Mary is?

4. What are some of the risks to a client when hospitalization is needed? How would you assess this?

5. While you are working in the emergency room a client is admitted with abdominal pain. He tells you that he has recently been diagnosed with TB. Would the precautions you use with this client differ from the precautions used with other clients in the ER? Explain your rationale.

6. Another client comes in with a deep laceration in his right thigh, the result of a motorcycle accident. You open up a sterile kit to clean and dress the wound. You realize that you need more sponges. What would you do to get them? Explain your rationale.

7. The client with the lacerated thigh tells you that he is not sure when he had his last tetanus shot but it was a long time ago. The physician orders a tetanus booster to be given IM. In preparing the medication you should follow what guidelines?

8.   What are your responsibilities after administering the tetanus booster?

9.   When a client is receiving an intravenous infusion, what is the nurse's responsibility regarding the IV site?

10. In the immediate postoperative stage, clients are carefully monitored until their physiological status is stabilized. What does this monitoring consist of?

■ ENRICHMENT ACTIVITIES

1.   With a friend, discuss several things that each of you do to fulfill the requirements of Clark's model of a wellness life-style: eating well, being fit, feeling good, caring for self and others, fitting in, and being responsible. Identify areas where you feel you have established healthy habits. In what areas do you feel you could improve?

2.   Consider the areas in which you feel you could improve. In reflecting upon your pattern of behavior, can you identify any events that might be associated with and possibly contributing to the behavior? List as many self-management strategies as you can for eliminating the behavior that should be changed and establishing a new, healthier pattern.

3.   Think about the various aspects of the environment you live in--your school environment, work environment, home environment. Evaluate each aspect for its contribution to a wellness life-style. Consider such things as the food and drinks available in the vending machines you use and the restaurants you frequent, the cleanliness and sanitation of institutional facilities, and opportunity and facilities for exercise that are available to you, municipal ordinances on smoking and drinking. How would you rate your environment for its contributions to wellness promotion?

4.   What precautions do you take in storing medications in your home? What do you do to keep medicines out of the way of children? Are you careful to discard outdated medicines or medicines without labels? To avoid using drugs that were prescribed for others? Think of several ways that medications might be hazardous in the home environment. Make a list of as many strategies as you can think of to minimize the potential hazards associated with the storage and use of medicine in the home.

5.   Think about your home as a biological environment. What are the reservoirs of bacterial contamination and infection in your home? What do you do to control or eliminate those reservoirs? Think about the ways you manage garbage or trash; clean the kitchen and bathroom; eliminate insects and pests. What practices do you engage in to prevent the spread of infection from one person to another?

■ SELF-EXAMINATION QUESTIONS

1.   State four major implications of a wellness life-style for eating well.

2.   State five major benefits of regular exercise.

3.   Which of the following is *not* an aspect of hardiness as defined by Kobasa?
     A. control (a belief that one can influence life events)
     B. commitment (a sense of purpose that promotes a desire to be actively involved in life-events)
     C. challenge (a belief that change is to be expected in life and should be welcomed as an opportunity for growth)
     D. caring (a belief that personal strength derives from a concern for others)

4.   List several emotional and physical signs of altered wellness.

5.   List three habits that are indicative of a lack of self-responsibility.

6.   List several stressors that are associated with admission to the hospital.

7.   Identify all of the alterations and potential alterations of well-being related to having surgery that you can think of.

CHAPTER 23

Self-expression

■ **BEHAVIORAL OBJECTIVES**

After studying this chapter, you should be able to:

1. Define self-expression.

2. State the importance of self-expression to health and well-being.

3. Discuss three functions of self-expression.

4. Discuss the concept of self-expression in relation to identity, self-concept, life structure, sexuality, and development.

5. Identify common modes of self-expression observed in everyday life.

6. State the importance of self-presentation and self-disclosure to self-expression.

7. State several characteristics of optimal self-expression.

8. Describe the impact of life change, illness, and loss on self-expression and state the implications for nursing practice.

9. Describe the grieving process.

10. Outline components of the client history and examination pertinent to assessing self-expression.

11. Outline nursing diagnoses related to self-expression, listing etiologies and defining characteristics.

12. Discuss nursing implementation related to self-expression for clients undergoing self-concept or body image changes, clients with concerns about sexuality, grieving clients, and dying clients.

13.   Discuss the collaborative role of the nurse in assisting clients with self-expression problems.

■ **KEY TERMS**

algor mortis	grief	rigor mortis
ambivalence	hope	self-disclosure
anticipatory grief	insight	self-expression
bereavement	livor mortis	self-presentation
catharsis	loneliness	sex
denial of illness	loss	sexuality
depersonalization	mourning	sexual orientation
distress	reference groups	situated identities
distress disclosure		

■ **REVIEW QUESTIONS**

Allison and Bill Chu have been married for five years. Allison, who is seven months pregnant, works as a nurse three evenings a week in the emergency room of the local community hospital. Bill works as a policeman during the day and is going to law school at night. They have a 3-year-old daughter, Jenny, who is cared for by Allison's mother, Betty, when Allison is at work.

1.   Self-expression comes from the concept of self, what the individual thinks, what others think, and the roles they play. List three roles for each of the people in the Chu family.

2.   When Allison comes for prenatal care, you, as her nurse, try to develop "therapeutic reciprocity" with her. Discuss what this means to nursing care.

3.   List the factors that affect self-expression.

Allison's father, Ed, died a year ago. It was not a complete surprise because Ed had heart problems, but it was still a hard loss to accept. Allison hopes she has a boy so she can name him after her father.

4.   Outline the grieving process and state where you think Allison is in this process.

5. Betty and Ed had been married thirty-five years. In view of Ed's recent death, you may want to assess Betty for any disturbances in self-esteem. What does this mean and what would you look for?

6. In the course of your conversation with Betty, she mentions that she and Ed used to go square dancing and that she misses it. She asks you whether you think it would be awful of her to try and find another partner to go with. What would you consider in your response to Betty?

7. In helping Allison and Bill prepare for the birth of their baby, why is it important to discuss Jenny and what her reaction might be to the new baby?

8. A client's first hospitalization experience may precipitate a crisis of self-esteem and impair self-expression. What should the nurse do to avoid or minimize this?

9. What are some of the needs the nurse must be aware of in caring for a client who is chronically ill?

10. Discuss how a nurse should relate to a client who is angry.

■ **ENRICHMENT ACTIVITIES**

1. Situated identities are identities that reside in the relationship between persons and their environments and are "fixed" by an individual's connections to particular other people. Make a list of the important people in your life. Next to each name, write your relationship and the role you play with respect to that person. For example, you may be Audrey's friend, Scott's sister, and so on. List as many names and corresponding identities as you can. From this list of situated identities, develop another list of "definitions of me" that correspond; for example, "I am a good friend," "I am a pesky sister." Rank these concepts of self in order of priority according to how important each is to your self-esteem. (Think about what your life would be like if suddenly certain roles became impossible, or certain identities were lost.) Which roles are central? Which are not so important?

2. People define their selves in evaluative, even judgmental, terms. These self-evaluations are the basis for self-esteem and represent a subjective estimate of how close one approaches one's self-ideal. Think about one or two of your close friends. Make a list of a few of their best qualities. Which ones do you think they are aware of? How do you know? What behavior indicates their awareness? Ask your friends to write their own lists. Compare your list with theirs. How well do they match?

3. Depression is a symptom of diminished well-being and is a common reaction to events that alter one's self-concept in a way that reduces self-esteem. Think about the people you know who have experienced depression. How did you know they were depressed? Make a list of the various outward signs that you observed. What were the feelings they experienced? Can you identify differences in the behavioral patterns of depression you observed. Have you ever been depressed? In what ways did your feelings and behavior change?

■ **SELF-EXAMINATION QUESTIONS**

1. Define self-expression.

2. Distinguish between the public self and the private self.

3. What aspects of self-expression are manifested in life structure and patterns of one's life?

4. What is the relationship of choices and choice making to self-expression?

5. Which of the following are *not* functions of self-expression?
    A. communicating self-identity
    B. assisting others
    C. establishing interpersonal relationships
    D. being responsible
    E. coping

6. State the relationship between caring and self-expression.

7. How is distress disclosure analogous to a fever?

8. Define catharsis.

9. List the phases of the sexual response.

10. Define what is meant by the "denial of illness."

11. Distinguish betwen bereavement, grief, and mourning.

CHAPTER 24

Skin and Tissue Integrity

■ **BEHAVIORAL OBJECTIVES**

After studying this chapter, you should be able to:

1. Discuss at least three functions of skin and mucosa.

2. Name at least four factors that influence skin and tissue integrity and describe their effects.

3. Discuss three examples of altered skin and mucosal integrity.

4. Describe the difference between primary and secondary skin lesions and list three examples of each.

5. Describe four types of wounds.

6. Discuss two processes in each of the phases of wound healing.

7. Compare and contrast healing by primary and secondary intention.

8. Discuss a collaborative approach to a health history specific to skin and tissue.

9. Describe the main elements of a skin and tissue examination.

10. State five examples of etiologies of impaired skin and tissue integrity according to the taxonomy of nursing diagnoses.

11. Discuss three examples of nursing implementation for impaired skin and tissue integrity for each of the following levels of care: preventive, supportive, restorative, and rehabilitative.

12. Discuss the importance of collaborative nurse-client management of skin and tissue integrity.

13. Discuss four general nursing approaches to enhance wound healing.

■ KEY TERMS

buccal mucosa	exudate	plaque
caries	fibroblast	pressure ulcer
collagen	gingiva	primary intention healing
conjunctiva	gingivitis	primary lesion
contusion	granulation tissue	rhinitis
cornea	hematoma	sclera
cyanosis	hemorrhage	secondary intention healing
debride	incision	secondary lesion
dehiscence	inflammation	shearing
dermatitis	ischemia	stomatitis
dermis	laceration	subcutaneous fat
ecchymosis	lesion	tartar
emollient	macrophage	thrombus
epidermis	normal flora	urethritis
epithelialization	phagocytosis	vaginitis
erythema	pharyngitis	wound
eschar	pilomotor activity	

■ REVIEW QUESTIONS

Martin Silk, a 22-year-old college student, came to the student health center because of a burn he sustained on the inner aspect of his leg. He said he got it from the exhaust pipe on his motorcycle. Your first step is assessment of his wound.

1. What is the difference between first-, second-, and third-degree burns?

2. It is your job to teach Martin how to care for his burn. He needs to keep it clean and prevent infection. What are the cardinal signs and symptoms of inflammation?

3. Martin has an appointment to come back in two days to find out whether the wound is healing properly. Describe the process of wound healing.

4. Martin is young and healthy so his wound should heal well. What factors might impair wound healing in infants and small children?

5. Assessing skin lesions for proper management is a mutual nurse-client function. What are some of the areas to explore for assessment and teaching?

6. List the nursing diagnoses of skin and tissue integrity.

7. One of the most important things a nurse does for a client is to promote optimum skin and tissue integrity. When the client is bed-ridden, in the hospital or the home, a bed bath is especially important. Discuss the bed bath procedure and its importance.

8. Gloves are used when changing wound dressings. Explain when you would use them and who they are protecting.

9. What is the purpose of a wound culture and when is it obtained?

10. Nursing researchers have studied the care of pressure ulcers. What do the findings mean to a nurse?

■ ENRICHMENT ACTIVITIES

1. Make a list of all of the substances that your skin is exposed to on a regular basis. Include all of the various personal and household cleaning products you use; for example, hand soaps, dish soaps, laundry soaps, bleaches. Check the labels of these products for a listing of active ingredients. What chemicals do they contain? Are

the ingredients identified? Are any of them potentially irritating to the skin? Are there warnings on the labels? Do the labels specify what to do if exposure results in skin irritation? What is your opinion about the adequacy of product labeling? Consider the lotions you use. Do any of them contain alcohol? What precautions do you take to protect your skin from exposure to harmful chemicals?

2. The deterioration of Earth's ozone layer has been in the news lately. Fluorocarbon-containing materials such as refrigerants and some propellants are thought to be responsible for the widening hole in the ozone layer. The ozone layer is important because it filters harmful solar rays that can produce skin cancer. Talk to several of your friends and acquaintances. Ask them what they know about the importance of the ozone layer. Do their responses indicate that they are sensitive to the potential environmental and personal danger that the loss of ozone represents?

3. Talk to several of your friends about their use of sunscreens. Ask them why they do or do not use it, and who they think should use sunscreen. Ask them about their sunbathing practices. Do they use sunscreen at the beach or swimming pool?

4. Other than chemicals, list the hazards to the skin and skin integrity that exist in your home environment. Be sure to consider those hazards that might result in burns or wounds. What precautions do you take to prevent accidents that might harm the skin?

5. With a friend, examine each other for skin lesions. Write your findings down. Be sure to consider the location, distribution, pattern, and type of lesion. Is a freckle a lesion? What kind? Is a bruise a lesion? What kind?

■ SELF-EXAMINATION QUESTIONS

1. Which of the following is *not* a layer or structure of the skin?
   A. epidermis
   B. dermis
   C. mucosa
   D. subcutaneous fat
   E. eccrine glands

2. List three components of the dermis.

3. List five functions of the skin and mucosa.

4. Which of the following is *not* an expected skin variation of the neonate?
   A. lanugo
   B. milia
   C. petechiae
   D. mongolian spot
   E. capillary hemangiomas
   F. dermatitis
   G. jaundice

5. Name six vitamins that are likely to result in skin disease when deficient in an individual's daily diet.

6. Which of the following is *not* generally considered to be a tooth and gum problem?
A. plaque
B. pruritis
C. caries
D. gingivitis
E. tartar

7. Differentiate between an ecchymosis and a hematoma.

8. What is "epithelialization"?

9. Describe healing by secondary intention.

10. Which of the following is *not* a complication of wound healing?
A. eschar
B. hemorrhage
C. infection
D. separation
E. keloids

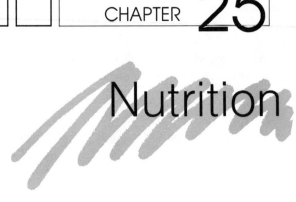

CHAPTER 25

Nutrition

■ **BEHAVIORAL OBJECTIVES**

After studying this chapter, you should be able to:

1. Discuss the role of nutrition in the prevention of illness, restoration of health, and promotion of high-level wellness.

2. Define energy balance and identify the factors influencing energy input and output in the human energy system.

3. Define how to calculate the total daily energy requirement for a given client.

4. Describe the processes that are involved in the digestion and absorption of food.

5. Describe how the metabolism of carbohydrates, proteins, and fats occurs in the human system.

6. Describe the cultural dimensions of a client's nutritional needs, and discuss why nurses must consider these in assessing and planning care.

7. Describe the following guidelines and standards available to assist in nutritional planning: Recommended Dietary Allowances, four food groups, and Senate Select Committee Recommendations.

8. Describe the etiology and symptoms of selected nutritional deficiency diseases.

9. Outline the components of the nutritional history and suggest questions to obtain the needed information.

10. List and describe physical examination procedures useful to assess nutritional status.

11. Identify diagnostic tests that contribute information relevant to a nutritional assessment.

12. Identify at least three nursing diagnoses from the North American Nursing Diagnosis Association (NANDA) taxonomy that relate to nutritional problems.

13. Identify subjective and objective data suggestive of each diagnosis.

14. Describe nursing implementation appropriate for alleviating nutritional alterations.

15. Describe the importance of collaboration for optimum nutrition among the nurse, the client, and the dietitian, including the appropriate roles that can be taken by each.

■ KEY TERMS

absorption
amino acid
anabolism
anorexia nervosa
bulimia
cachexia
carbohydrate
catabolism
chyme
complementary protein
complete protein
complex carbohydrate
dietary fiber
digestion
energy balance
enteral

essential amino acid
essential nutrient
fat
fatty acid
gluconeogenesis
glycogen
glycogenolysis
insulin
intrinsic factor
kilocalorie
kwashiorkor
lipid
marasmus
metabolism
mineral
monounsaturated fatty acid

nitrogen balance
nutrient
nutrition
obesity
overweight
peristalsis
polyunsaturated fatty acid
protein
protein-calorie malnutrition
Recommended Dietary
    Allowances
Recommended Nutrient Intakes
saturated fatty acid
simple carbohydrate
starch
total parenteral nutrition
vitamin

■ REVIEW QUESTIONS

1. Define energy balance and identify several factors that influence energy input and energy output in the human energy system.

2. List and describe the six major classes of nutrients.

3. Define:

digestion

absorption

metabolism

4. Discuss five factors that affect a client's nutritional status.

5. Define the following nutritional disorders:

kwashiorkor

marasmus

protein deficiency state

cachexia

anorexia

bulimia

obesity

6. Mrs. Kramer is fifty pounds overweight. List five questions to be included in her nutritional assessment. List some areas of importance during the nutritional examination.

7. Mrs. Kramer's nursing diagnosis is Altered Nutrition: More than Body Requirements. Cite a general etiology related to this diagnosis. List several risk factors for excess caloric intake relative to metabolic need.

8. Mrs. Clemons, 67 years old, is a retired school teacher and wife. Discuss some practical advice you might give her to help her reduce her food expenditure and the effort required by her to prepare her meals.

9. Mr. Silver, 59 years old, has been in the hospital for three days for a variety of tests. He says he is not really hungry. List some nursing strategies to help him improve his appetite. During Mr. Silver's hospitalization he is placed on a variety of diets. Explain when a regular, soft, liquid, and clear hospital diet is typically used.

10. Mr. Silver is diagnosed with cancer of the colon and undergoes a colostomy. List some nursing strategies to maximize his nutritional status after this acute episode.

■ ENRICHMENT ACTIVITIES

1. Take a food that contains protein, fat, and carbohydrate (for example, a hamburger) and trace the digestion, absorption, and metabolism of each of its nutrients.

2. Keep a 24-hour diary of your own diet. With the data collected, analyze your daily diet for its caloric and nutritional adequacy in relation to your daily energy expenditure and the RDAs.

3. Keep a record of your family's weekly food shopping. Analyze the foods that have been purchased for accordance with the principles of good nutrition discussed in this chapter. Identify any changes in food purchasing that would result in a healthier dietary pattern. Also, identify any food purchases that could be altered to decrease the amount of money spent, without sacrificing the quality of the diet.

4. Design a day's menu that would be in maximum accordance with the principles of good nutrition.

■ SELF-EXAMINATION QUESTIONS

1. Mrs. Clark, a 30-year-old, 5'5" housewife, is trying to lose weight in time for her summer vacation. She consults a nurse in a nearby clinic for advice. She has no health problems other than being 20 pounds overweight. What is an appropriate response by the nurse?
   A. Refer her to a dietician.
   B. Tell her to go on a high-protein, low-carbohydrate diet for 2 months.
   C. Tell her to begin a program of regular exercise.
   D. Tell her to limit her daily caloric intake to 500 kcal.

2. Mr. Norberto comes from a family with a long history of heart disease. His serum lipids, triglycerides, and cholesterol are well above normal. He is trying to limit his intake of fats and cholesterol completely. What advice should the nurse give him about an appropriate diet?
   A. He should include some monounsaturated fats in his diet.
   B. He should limit only polyunsaturated fats.
   C. He is doing the right thing.
   D. He should avoid pasta and other starchy foods.

3. An infant is brought to the emergency room, having been found abandoned in the street. He is extremely thin but has a distended abdomen and peripheral edema. The nurse should suspect that this infant has which of the following nutritional diseases?
   A. scurvy
   B. rickets
   C. pellagra
   D. kwashiorkor

4. Referring to the infant in question 3, which of the following diagnostic tests would confirm the nurse's impression?
   A. lymphocyte count
   B. serum albumin
   C. hemoglobin
   D. all of the above
   E. none of the above

5. Mr. Wu had a laryngectomy 3 days ago.   His physician orders a tube feeling schedule of Ensure, 250 mL, to be given every 4 hours.   One hour after the first feeding, Mr. Wu begins to have severe diarrhea.   Which of the following nursing measures is appropriate?
   A. Recognize this as a normal response and reassure Mr. Wu of this.
   B. Discuss with the physician changing the feedings to continuous administration.
   C. Administer only half the dose at the next feeding.
   D. Give a different formula at the next feeding.

6. A 24-year-old lactovegetarian client is admitted to the hospital for surgical removal of an ovarian cyst.   What advice is most appropriate for the nurse to give her about her diet after discharge?
   A. Eat more eggs.
   B. Eat more chicken.
   C. Eat more beans and nuts.
   D. Eat more fish.

CHAPTER 26

Elimination

■ **BEHAVIORAL OBJECTIVES**

After studying this chapter, you should be able to:

1. Name and describe the primary function of the major organs of bowel and urinary elimination.

2. Describe the normal patterns of elimination in an adult.

3. List four factors affecting bowel function and four factors affecting urinary function and describe their consequences.

4. Describe variations in elimination that may occur in the course of the life cycle.

5. Identify six alterations in bowel elimination.

6. Identify five alterations in urinary elimination.

7. List data to be obtained in an elimination history.

8. Identify essential elements of a nursing examination of bowel and urinary function.

9. Identify at least six diagnostic tests used in determining elimination status.

10. List three nursing diagnoses describing altered bowel elimination and identify an etiology for each.

11. List six nursing diagnoses describing altered urinary elimination and identify an etiology for each.

12. Describe two examples of preventive, supportive, restorative, and rehabilitative nursing implementation that promote bowel and bladder function and give the rationale for each.

13. Describe common learning needs of clients with an alteration in elimination.

14.   Write a client care plan for a client with altered elimination.

15.   Discuss the nurse's role in collaborating with the client to promote optimal elimination function.

■   **KEY TERMS**

adynamic ileus	fecal incontinence	paralytic ileus
anuria	flatulence	peristalsis
constipation	functional incontinence	polyuria
diarrhea	gastrocolic reflex	proteinuria
duodenocolic reflex	glomerular filtration rate	stoma
dysuria	Kegel exercises	stress incontinence
elimination	melena	urinary frequency
enema	nephron	urinary incontinence
enuresis	nocturia	urinary retention
fecal impaction	oliguria	Valsalva maneuver

■   **REVIEW QUESTIONS**

1.   A 20-year-old woman arrives at the health center complaining of vomiting and diarrhea during the past 24 hours.   She cannot eat anything without vomiting and feels very weak.   What elimination data should be collected during the nursing assessment?

2.   What measurements will provide information about the elimination status in this woman?

3.   What general observations should be gathered when examining this woman?

4.   To verify the significance of the general observations, what additional data should the nurse collect?

5.   Mr. Martinez, a 78-year-old man who lives alone and has no living family members, complains of decreased number of stools that are hard and are causing him to have painful bowel movements. According to the article by McShane and McLane on page 1153 of your text, ("Is Constipation a Single Entity or Are There Different Types?"), what type of constipation does Mr. Martinez have?

6. List possible etiologies of Mr. Martinez' problems according to McShane and McLane.

7. Joe Brown, 18 years old, was in an automobile accident. He is a candidate for a bowel training program. He has control of his abdominal muscles and his anal sphincter. List the components of a bowel training program.

8. Joe must learn how to do self-catheterization. He has an intact voiding reflex arc but no sensory input from the bladder. List important points to include when teaching self-catheterization.

9. How would you evaluate the results of Joe's bowel and bladder training?

■ ENRICHMENT ACTIVITIES

1. One of your friends recently had an ileostomy. Identify resources in your community that could be helpful to your friend. List services that these resources can provide. Compare your list of available services with the lists of other students.

2. Identify factors in your life that could promote or hinder urine elimination. Keep a record of your own fluid intake and output for 24 hours. State how your intake affected your urinary elimination. Describe alterations in normal patterns of urine elimination you have experienced.

3. Identify factors in your life that could promote or hinder bowel elimination. Keep a record of your own fluid and food intake and output for 24 hours. State how this can affect bowel elimination. Describe alterations in normal patterns of bowel elimination you have experienced.

4. A relative is bedridden at home and needs to use a bedpan. Where can the family purchase a bedpan? Describe how you would collaborate with the client and family to help them learn the appropriate use of the bedpan.

5. Your neighbor is home from the hospital after having a colostomy. What type of life-style changes does your neighbor face? How can an enterostomal therapist be helpful? Where can your neighbor obtain ostomy appliances?

■ SELF-EXAMINATION QUESTIONS

1. Is each of the following questions true (T) or false (F)?

   _____ (1)   Prolonged use of laxatives may cause the large intestine to be less responsive to laxatives.

   _____ (2)   A person with a colostomy will generally have more liquid stool than a person with an ileostomy.

   _____ (3)   An ostomy is an artificial opening through the abdominal wall.

   _____ (4)   The presence of blood in the stool is a normal occurrence.

2. Match the terms in column A with the appropriate definitions in column B.

<u>A</u>		<u>B</u>
_____ (1) anuria	a.	urine in bladder after voiding
_____ (2) micturition	b.	inability to control stool or urine flow
_____ (3) residual urine	c.	lack of urine production
_____ (4) incontinence	d.	urine production of less than 30 ml per hour
_____ (5) oliguria	e.	urination

3. List five possible etiologies for the nursing diagnosis of constipation.

4. All of the following are possible etiologies for diarrhea *except*:
   A. intestinal irritation.
   B. emotional stress.
   C. chronic use of enemas and laxatives.
   D. high-osmolality nutrition formulas.

5. The most important part of preventive care for elimination concerns is _____.

6. Exercise is an important part of supportive care for mild constipation because exercise _____

   _____.

CHAPTER 27

Oxygenation

■ **BEHAVIORAL OBJECTIVES**

After studying this chapter, you should be able to:

1. Discuss the major organs involved in each of the following processes: ventilation, diffusion, perfusion, and cellular respiration.

2. Define and describe the processes of ventilation, diffusion, perfusion, and cellular respiration.

3. Discuss the impact of general health, development, and the environment on oxygenation.

4. Discuss at least two factors that cause alterations in ventilation, diffusion, perfusion, and cellular respiration.

5. Discuss how these factors can cause hypoventilation, hyperventilation, or tissue necrosis.

6. List data that are important in an oxygenation history.

7. Describe essential elements of an oxygenation examination.

8. List at least five laboratory tests or diagnostic examinations relevant to oxygenation.

9. Define three nursing diagnoses describing altered oxygenation and identify and explain at least two etiologies for each nursing diagnosis.

10. Describe at least two examples of nursing implementation for preventive, supportive, restorative, and rehabilitative oxygenation care.

11. Discuss nurses' responsibilities associated with oxygen administration.

12. Identify strategies to evaluate effectiveness of nursing implementation to support oxygenation.

13. Write a client care plan to promote optimum oxygenation for a specific client.

■ **KEY TERMS**

anatomical dead space	hyperventilation	splinting
atelectasis	hypoventilation	surfactant
diastole	hypoxia	sustained maximal inspiration
diffusion	inspiration	systole
expiration	inspiratory capacity	tachypnea
expiratory reserve volume	inspiratory reserve volume	tidal volume
functional residual capacity	oxygenation	total lung capacity
hematocrit	perfusion	ventilation
hemoglobin	residual volume	vital capacity
hyperpnea		

■ **REVIEW QUESTIONS**

1. Define and describe the following terms.

   ventilation

   diffusion

   perfusion

2. Discuss life-style factors that affect oxygenation in healthy individuals.

3. Mrs. Duxbury, 76 years old, has come to the clinic for her yearly examination. Discuss the differences in anatomy and physiology related to oxygenation at her age.

4. List the signs and symptoms of hyperventilation and hypoventilation.

5. Define the following terms.

    hypoxia

    hypercapnia

    hypocapnia

    tissue necrosis

6. Mrs. Davis is a single professional woman complaining of wheezing and tightness in the chest. Describe the health history you would obtain related to oxygenation.

7. Mrs. Jones, 46 years old, started smoking when she was 20. She has smoked one pack a day until 2 years ago when she began smoking 2 packs a day. What is her pack-year history?

    At this time Mrs. Jones does not have any symptoms of poor oxygenation. What role does the nurse have in relation to Mrs. Jones' smoking habit?

8. Mr. King will be undergoing abdominal surgery.   What nursing care given before surgery can prevent postoperative oxygenation problems?

9. Mr. Weinberg was admitted to the hospital in respiratory distress. Describe the nursing actions that will reduce oxygen demands in this client.

Mr. Weinberg is receiving oxygen via nasal prongs. Discuss the nurse's responsibility related to oxygen therapy.

10. Mr. Su, 56, has smoked since he was 14 and has been a 4-pack-a-day smoker for the last 10 years. He has chronic obstructive lung disease, a chronic oxygenation dysfunction.   List the topics you would include in a client education program for Mr. Su.

■ ENRICHMENT ACTIVITIES

1. Watch the newspapers and local magazines in your area for two weeks for stories related to people with oxygenation problems. What causes were identified? Were life-style factors involved? Were some causes accidental? Was emergency treatment required? Judging from these stories, does your community have effective services for handling such problems?

2. Talk to several people you know who are not health care professionals. Ask them if they have received training in cardiopulmonary resuscitation (CPR). Have they ever been in a situation where they felt they needed skill in CPR? Have you? Should every citizen be taught CPR?   Why or why not? Discuss this questions with a classmate.

3. You have just been notified that a member of your family has a serious, chronic problem with oxygenation and will need oxygen therapy at home. How might this change things in your home? What tasks might have to be reassigned? Would your house or apartment present barriers to the use of oxygen equipment? What hazards might be introduced by the use of oxygen? Does anyone in your home smoke? If so, what problems would that pose?

4. Talk to people you know who smoke. Ask them for their opinions about the health risks associated with smoking and with passive smoke. How do they feel about the increasing restrictions on smokers? What are their feelings about quitting? Have they tried? What were the obstacles?

■ **SELF-EXAMINATION QUESTIONS**

1. The role of surfactant includes all of the following *except*:
   A. decreased surface tension.
   B. increased ciliary action.
   C. increased alveolar stability.
   D. help keep alveoli dry.

2. You are a nurse in a physician's office. A client who is a heavy smoker is having abdominal surgery in four weeks. What do you tell the client regarding his smoking?
   A. Quit now; natural respiratory defenses will help rid your lungs of the products of smoking, which will help prevent respiratory complications.
   B. Do nothing; four weeks is not enough time to improve your respiratory condition.
   C. Stop the day before surgery; preoperative deep-breathing exercises will help you rid your lungs of sputum.

3. A client is to have a bronchoscopy. She and her family should be told all of the following *except*:
   A. the client will be NPO before the procedure.
   B. local medication will be given to reduce the gag reflex.
   C. the client will be asked to cough during the procedure.
   D. no sedatives are given so that the client can cooperate during the procedure.
   E. no food or drink is given following the procedure until the client's gag reflex returns.

4. The best way to assess the adequacy of a client's ventilation is to:
   A. watch the client breathe.
   B. ask the client whether he or she feels short of breath.
   C. assess exercise tolerance.
   D. assess PCO_2.
   E. assess PO_2.

5. Why is sedation contraindicated for a client who is in respiratory distress?
   A. The sedated client is unable to describe his or her symptoms.
   B. Sedative medications interact with respiratory medications.
   C. Sedatives depress the respiratory drive.
   D. Sedatives relax the respiratory muscles.

6. Match the terms in column A with the correct definitions in column B.

A	B
_____ (1) apnea	a. increase in the rate or depth of breathing
_____ (2) bradypnea	b. rapid, shallow breathing
_____ (3) dyspnea	c. decreased respiratory rate
_____ (4) hyperpnea	d. subjective sensation of shortness of breath
_____ (5) tachypnea	e. cessation of breathing

CHAPTER 28

Sleep–Rest Patterns

■ **BEHAVIORAL OBJECTIVES**

After studying this chapter, you should be able to:

1. Differentiate between the functions and characteristics of REM and NREM sleep.

2. List the consequences of REM sleep deprivation.

3. List the factors affecting sleep.

4. Summarize how sleep-rest patterns differ in each of the following age groups: infants, toddlers, children, adolescents, young adults, middle-aged adults, and older adults.

5. Describe at least five disorders of initiating and maintaining sleep found during the life cycle.

6. Describe at least two causes of excessive somnolence during the life cycle.

7. Describe at least three causes of disorders of arousal in individuals under 20 years of age.

8. State four causes of sleep problems in the elderly.

9. Explain the purpose of the following in assisting the client with sleep problems: polysomnography, sleep history, observation of the client, sleep nursing diagnosis, and sleep care plan.

10. State at least 10 nursing diagnoses related to the diagnosis of sleep-rest patterns.

11. List data to be obtained in a sleep-rest history.

12. List at least five nursing implementations useful in the promotion of sleep and rest.

13. Discuss the importance of collaboration in the management of sleep-rest problems.

■ **KEY TERMS**

ascending reticular activating
   system
fatigue
insomnia
narcolepsy

nocturnal myoclonus
nocturnal polysomnogram
nonrapid eye movement sleep
obstructive sleep apnea
parasomnias

rapid eye movement sleep
rest
sleep
sleep apnea
sundown syndrome

■ **REVIEW QUESTIONS**

1.   Discuss the differences between the functions and characteristics of REM and NREM sleep.

2.   List two consequences of REM sleep deprivation.

3.   List factors that affect sleep-rest patterns.

4.   List two causes of excessive somnolence in adults.

5.   List three causes of disorders of arousal (parasomnias) in individuals under 20 years of age.

6.   List four causes of sleep problem in the elderly.

7. For each of the following five categories, name two nursing diagnoses that can be related to sleep-rest patterns.

   physical

   emotional

   self-conceptual

   sociocultural

   sexual

8. List the data that should be collected for a sleep-rest history.

9. List four nursing implementations that can promote optimum sleep and rest.

10. Identify three major categories of sleep dysfunction.

■ ENRICHMENT ACTIVITIES

1. Keep a diary of your bedtime routines for one week. What time do you go to bed? What are the things you do to prepare for going to bed? How long does it take you to fall asleep? How many times do you awaken during the night? What are the things that cause you to awaken? What time do you awaken in the morning? How many total hours did you sleep? From your observations, would you say that your body rhythms are predictable? For example, do you become sleepy about the same time each day? Do you need an alarm clock to awaken, or do you tend to wake up on your own? Next time you go to bed, change your sleeping habits somewhat. For example, keep a light on in the room, or turn the radio on or off. Do you notice any difference in your sleep pattern? What is your overall feeling of being rested the next day?

2. Talk to a few friends and ask them about their nighttime sleep preparation routines. What routines are the same as or different from yours? Discuss instances in which each of you has had trouble falling asleep. What kinds of factors were responsible? Were there any commonalities? What role does stress play? What are some of the comfort measures that the group identifies--things that promote sleep and seem to help you rest?

3. Talk to several members of your family of different ages: include some children. Ask them about their sleep preparation routines. Do interruptions in their nightly routines disturb their sleep? Ask them about the effect of having lights on or off, or of noise; about eating prior to bedtime or of toileting routines such as face washing, bathing, hair brushing, and so on. Do any of your relatives keep an irregular schedule? What things do they do to promote sleep?

4. What are the pros and cons of napping in the middle of the day? Ask friends or relatives about their napping habits. What is the effect of napping on their sleep routine? What do you think some of the pros and cons of client napping during the day might be? What are some factors to consider in constructing such a list?

■ SELF-EXAMINATION QUESTIONS

1. The consequences of REM sleep deprivation include all of the following *except*:
    A. apathy.
    B. irritability.
    C. increased pain sensitivity.
    D. increased alertness.

2. The usual progression of the sleep cycle is:
    A. Stage I, II, III, IV, REM, III, II, I.
    B. Stage I, II, III, IV, III, REM, II, I.
    C. Stage I, II, III, IV, III, II, REM, II.
    D. Stage I, II, REM, III, IV, III, II.

3. As one ages which of the following sleep changes occur?
    A. Sleep onset latency decreases, and there is more total sleep time.
    B. Nocturnal awakenings decrease and total sleep time increases.
    C. Nocturnal awakenings increase and sleep onset latency decreases.
    D. Sleep onset latency increases and total sleep time decreases.

4. Risk factors associated with disturbed sleep include all of the following *except*:
    A. vigorous exercise 6-8 hours before bedtime.
    B. vigorous exercise 1-2 hours before bedtime.
    C. regular use of alcohol before bedtime.
    D. regular use of sleeping medication before bedtime.

5. Which of the following is an appropriate nursing intervention for a toddler experiencing difficulty falling asleep?
    A. Suggest that the parents read to the child until sleep occurs.
    B. Suggest that the child fall asleep in a parent's lap.
    C. Suggest that the child go to bed at the same time each night.
    D. Suggest that the child be allowed to cry until sleep occurs.

6. Identify the common causes of sleep problems in the adolescent.

CHAPTER 29

Neurosensory Integration

■ **BEHAVIORAL OBJECTIVES**

After studying this chapter, you should be able to:

1. Describe functions served by neurosensory integration.

2. Identify and describe the anatomical components, pathways, and components and the physiological mechanisms involved in pain.

3. Discuss the importance of neurosensory integration for the collaborative nurse-client relationship.

4. Identify factors affecting neurosensory integration.

5. Identify protective structures and processes involved in neurosensory functioning.

6. List and describe the basic causes of neurosensory alterations.

7. List and describe alterations in consciousness, memory, speech and language, and movement.

8. Describe alterations in perception, emotion, and memory.

9. Identify essential components of a neurosensory history and examination.

10. Explain the purpose of selected neurological diagnostic tests.

11. State three nursing diagnoses for clients experiencing an alteration in neurosensory integration.

12. Identify appropriate nursing implementations that reflect preventive, supportive, restorative, and rehabilitative levels of care for clients experiencing alterations in neurosensory integration.

■ KEY TERMS

affect
anesthesia
aphasia
arousal
central vision
classical conditioning
cognition
communication
consciousness
content
emotion
feeling

habituation
hyperesthesia
hypoesthesia
immediate memory
involuntary movement
language
long-term memory
memory
mood
movement
neurons
pain

paresthesia
perception
peripheral vision
sensitization
sensory deprivation
sensory overload
short-term memory
speech
thought
tone
voluntary movement

■ REVIEW QUESTIONS

1. List the three components of the pain response.

2. List the three types of memory.

3. List the factors that affect neurosensory integration.

4. Define the following terms commonly used to describe alterations in consciousness:

    alert

    confused

    delirious

    obtunded

stuporous

semi-consciousness

coma

deep coma

5. List five questions that should be answered during a neurosensory assessment.

6. Describe the Glascow Coma Scale.

7. The students in your class have been invited to participate in a health education program on your campus. Describe the topics you would want to include in the program in relation to safety issues and accident prevention.

8. List the supportive care related to enhancing clients' vision.

9. Describe the nursing observations of a client who is having a seizure.

10. List the approaches that are available to assist a client who has chronic pain.

■ **ENRICHMENT ACTIVITIES**

1. Tie a blindfold around your eyes and keep it in place for a 15-minute period. Continue your normal activities. Afterward write down the ways you adapted to the problems you confronted. How did you deal with barriers to mobility? What problems did you have in accomplishing skilled activities such as writing? What senses did you employ in an attempt to compensate?

2. Head and spinal cord injuries are serious public health problems that can be prevented by wearing helmets while riding bicycles and motorcycles and other open vehicles and by using automobile airbags. What are the laws in your state pertaining to these practices? What political interest groups are involved in shaping your state's policies on the prevention of head and spinal cord injuries?

3. From time to time, everyone is a victim of sensory overload. List situations in which your senses have been bombarded to the point that you experienced stress. Describe your behavior. What did you do to reduce the stress? Compare your list and behavior description to those of a friend. Did you list similar experiences? What role does age play in the experience of sensory overload?

4. Think of an experience you have had with pain. What did you do to relieve the pain? What does your family commonly rely on for pain relief? Do you use medications for pain relief? Are they always effective? Do you try other things before taking medication? List some non-pharmaceutical means that you have used for pain relief. What role did environmental stimuli such as noise play in aggravating your pain and what role did reducing or eliminating those stimuli play in getting relief from pain?

5. Memory is very important to adapting and coping in daily life. All of us forget things from time to time. How have other people assisted you in situations in which you have forgotten something important? What are some non-helpful things that others did? Think of the last time you misplaced your car keys. What memory aids

did you use to find them? What memory aids do you use to avoid forgetting things? Would any of these strategies help clients remember important things, such as taking their medications?

■ SELF-EXAMINATION QUESTIONS

1. List two components of consciousness and state their significance.

2. The vestibular apparatus is an important sensory reception center. Which of the following senses does the vestibular apparatus serve?
    A. pain
    B. vision
    C. balance
    D. tactile
    E. vibration

3. List the components of memory. Which component holds items of information for several minutes to hours?

4. List several mental activities that are involved in thought.

5. Distinguish between speech and language.

6. List several factors that are important in appraising the client's experience of pain.

7. Distinguish among spasticity, flaccidity, and rigidity--three states of resistance to passive muscle movement.

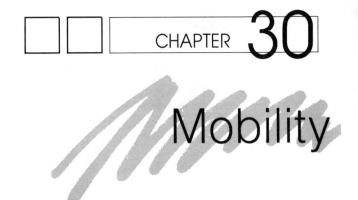

CHAPTER 30

Mobility

■ BEHAVIORAL OBJECTIVES

After studying this chapter, you should be able to:

1. Describe how each of the following affect mobility: musculoskeletal functioning, cardiopulmonary functioning, metabolic efficiency, and emotional status.

2. Briefly summarize the physiological response to increased muscular activity.

3. List and define the four components of fitness, and describe the type of activity required for optimum development of each component.

4. List at least six benefits of regular aerobic exercise and explain how exercise brings about these effects.

5. State two risks associated with exercise.

6. Describe how age, disability, general health, self-concept, and values affect mobility.

7. Describe at least three examples of problems in each of the following functional dimensions that result from decreased mobility: activity/mobility, rest/sleep, oxygenation, nutrition, fluid and elimination, sexuality, and psychological dimensions.

8. Describe essential elements of a mobility history.

9. Describe essential elements of a mobility examination.

10. Name three diagnostic tests useful in diagnosing mobility problems.

11. Define four nursing diagnoses that describe altered mobility.

12. Identify and explain at least two etiologies of each of the above diagnoses.

13. Describe at least three examples of preventive, supportive, restorative, and rehabilitative nursing implementation to promote, maintain, or enhance mobility.

14. List and explain seven basic guidelines for effective body mechanics.

■ **KEY TERMS**

active range of motion
activities of daily living
aerobic exercise
anaerobic glycolysis
antagonist
dangling
disuse phenomenon
disuse syndrome
eggcrate mattress overlay
endurance
exercise tolerance

fitness
flexibility
footboard
hand roll
heel and elbow protectors
isokinetic exercise
isometric exercise
isotonic exercise
orthostatic (postural)
    hypotension

passive range of motion
pressure reduction device
pressure relief bed
prosthesis
strength
synergist
trochanter roll
Valsalva maneuver

■ **REVIEW QUESTIONS**

1. List the components of fitness.

2. List the factors that affect mobility.

3. Define the following terms:

    aerobic exercise

    Valsalva maneuver

    isotonic exercise

    isometric exercise

    orthostatic hypotension

active range of motion exercises

activities of daily living (ADL)

4. Describe clients who are at high risk for developing pressure ulcers.

5. List the baseline data needed for assessing exercise tolerance.

6. What risk factors create a likelihood of developing disuse syndrome?

7. Discuss strategies that enhance a client's motivation to maintain an exercise program.

8. Mr. Thomas, 76, has Parkinson's disease, is confined to bed, and is being cared for at home by his daughter. List the guidelines that you will give to Mr. Thomas' daughter for effective protective body mechanics.

9. What protective devices can be used for Mr. Thomas (in his home) to maintain correct alignment and prevent pressure sores?

10. Discuss the implications of OBRA--the Omnibus Budget Reconciliation Act of 1987.

■ ENRICHMENT ACTIVITIES

1. Carry a notebook with you for one day and imagine as you move from place to place that your leg is in a large cast and you must use crutches. During the course of the day, envision and record the difficulties you encounter during your usual activities. For instance, would using crutches interfere with attending classes? What about work? How many stairs must you climb at home, school, or work? Do the stairs pose a problem? What about personal hygiene? Can you bathe, given the need to keep your cast dry? Which of your usual activities become impossible? At the end of the day, review your list of problems. What assistance would you require if the situation were real?

2. Interview someone with a permanent disability due to paralysis or muscle degeneration. What are the barriers to maintaining independence and mobility in daily life? How has the individual adapted to these barriers? Have changes in public services helped his or her adaptation? What changes in public services does this person want? What struggles have been experienced in achieving personal goals?

3. Identify a family member who is not as physically fit as he or she might be. What indicators do you observe? What accounts for the lack of fitness? Diet? Activity pattern? Other habits? Emotional or mental factors? Is your relative aware of his or her condition? Do any health beliefs interfere with fitness activities? What approach might help your relative to become more fit? What is your rationale?

■ SELF-EXAMINATION QUESTIONS

1. Which of the following statements is true of the ball-and-socket joint?

A. It is found at the knee and in the spine.

B. It allows for rotation movement only.

C. It is created by an ovoid bony projection that fits into an elliptical cavity.

D. It is involved in flexion-extension and adduction-abduction of the shoulder.

2.   Which of the following is *not* an effect of regular exercise?

A. resting heart rate decreases

B. pulmonary vital capacity expands

C. speed of neuromuscular impulse transmission accelerates

D. cholesterol transport to the liver may occur

3.   Which of the following is *not* an effect of immobility?

A. reduced stimulation of osteoblasts

B. reduced serum levels of low-density lipoproteins

C. carbon dioxide narcosis and respiratory acidosis

D. hypercalcemia

4.   The Romberg test is a test for:

A. range of motion.

B. balance.

C. tendon reflexes.

D. exercise tolerance.

5.   Which of the following is not a hazard associated with the use of Fowler's position?

A. reduced lung capacity

B. damage to skin over the scapulae and sacrum

C. shearing force and excessive pressure to the ischial tuberosities

D. thrombus formation due to pressure in the popliteal space.

CHAPTER 31

Fluid and Electrolyte Balance

■ **BEHAVIORAL OBJECTIVES**

After studying this chapter, you should be able to:

1. Define key terms associated with fluid, electrolyte, and acid-base balance.

2. Describe the physiological processes involved in the maintenance of fluid balance.

3. Discuss at least four variables that influence the movement of fluid between body fluid compartments.

4. State the quantities and functions of major electrolytes in body fluids and describe clinical manifestations of electrolyte imbalances.

5. Describe how the body maintains acid-base balance.

6. Identify the major buffering systems controlling acid-base balance.

7. Compare and contrast the four acid-base abnormalities.

8. Identify appropriate history questions designed to gain information regarding a client's fluid and electrolyte balance.

9. Describe health examination observations useful in assessing a client's fluid and electrolyte balance.

10. Identify the subjective and objective manifestations suggestive of fluid and electrolyte imbalances.

11. Identify the nursing diagnoses associated with fluid balance problems.

12. Specify nursing implementation designed to alleviate fluid and electrolyte imbalances.

13. Discuss the oral and parenteral replacement of fluids with respect to type, indications, maintenance, and discontinuation.

14. Discuss the nurse's role in collaborating with the client to promote, maintain, or restore body fluid, electrolyte, and acid-base balance.

■ KEY TERMS

anions	hypovolemia	pH
buffers	insensible loss	respiratory acidosis
cations	intravenous infusion	respiratory alkalosis
edema	isotonic	serum osmolality
hemolytic reaction	isotonic dehydration	shock
hypertonic	metabolic acidosis	third spacing
hypertonic dehydration	metabolic alkalosis	total body water
hypotonic	nasogastric gavage	total parenteral nutrition
hypotonic dehydration	obligatory urine output	venipuncture

■ REVIEW QUESTIONS

1. List six common functions of body fluids.

2. What factors affect fluid and electrolyte balance?

3. List the signs and symptoms and a cause of each of the following electrolyte alterations:

   hyponatremia

   hypernatremia

   hypokalemia

   hyperkalemia

hypocalcemia

hypercalcemia

hypomagnesemia

hypermagnesemia

hypophosphatemia

hyperphosphatemia

hypochloremia

hyperchloremia

4. Discuss the acid-base alterations associated with each of the following:

respiratory depression as a result of narcotic overdose

hyperventilation from anxiety

renal failure

excessive gastric suction

5. What general observations should the nurse include while performing a body fluid assessment?

6. Cite the possible significance of each of the following findings:

apathy, restlessness, apprehension

dry sticky mucous membranes

erythema and swelling of the tongue

crackles on auscultation

ascites

increased urine output

hyperactive deep tendon reflexes

muscle flaccidity

7. List several risk factors for fluid volume deficit.

8. Describe four strategies for identifying clients at risk for fluid imbalances.

9. Describe the nurse's role in treating fluid and electrolyte imbalances.

10. Mr. Lorden is receiving TPN therapy. What is the nurse's responsibility in providing safe and successful administration of TPN?

■ ENRICHMENT ACTIVITIES

1. Visit a fast food restaurant in your neighborhood. Ask for a list of the nutrient values of the items they serve. Using the list, total the sodium content for the menu items you buy. If you were on a sodium-restricted diet with a 1000 mg/d sodium limit, what entrees could you eat for breakfast or lunch without consuming your entire daily sodium allotment? What about a 500 mg/d sodium limit?

2. Keep a written record of your fluid intake and output for 3 days, whenever possible measuring instead of estimating and noting times and amounts. After completing the exercise, consider the difficulties you encountered in keeping the record. What inconveniences did you experience? Would any of them apply to a hospital setting? How did you feel about the procedure? Did they interfere in any way? What relationship did you find between your daily patterns of intake and output?

3. Imagine that someone important to you develops severe high blood pressure and requires a salt-restricted diet. You invite that person to dinner. Using a table of the nutrient values of common foods, plan a meal that contains no more that 750 mg sodium. What types of foods are relatively low in sodium content?

4. Try this simple home experiment. Take a stalk of celery. Divide the stalk into two approximately equal pieces. Fill two small plastic containers, approximately two cups in volume, with tap water. To one of the containers add two teaspoons of table salt. Cover both containers and place them in the refrigerator. Check the containers periodically, removing the stalks of celery and shaking them gently. What happens to the stalk in the salt solution? How does it compare in firmness to the stalk in the tap water? What physiochemical process does this illustrate? What conclusions can you draw about the concentration of the salt solution? What implications does this have for the care of clients?

5. Imagine that you have become dehydrated and that it becomes necessary for you to drink large volumes of fluid to regain your fluid balance. List some fluids that you believe might be appealing enough to drink in quantity. What fluids would you avoid? Why? What might happen if you drank coffee, tea, or colas on this regimen? What are the advantages of a beverage like Gatorade? Compare your list to that of a friend. Could you exchange lists and use each other's, or do you have individual preferences that might affect the success of a rehydration program?

■ SELF-EXAMINATION QUESTIONS

1. When the extracellular fluid becomes depleted, the kidneys respond by making:
   A. less urine.
   B. more urine.
   C. the usual amount of urine.
   D. dilute urine.

2. The process by which fluid moves from a red blood cell placed in a hypertonic fluid is known as:
   A. diffusion.
   B. active transport.
   C. osmosis.
   D. filtration.

3. Because of the loss of alkaline-rich intestinal fluid, prolonged diarrhea can lead to:
   A. respiratory acidosis.
   B. respiratory alkalosis.
   C. metabolic acidosis.
   D. metabolic alkalosis.

4. Which of the following is *not* a symptom of hypernatremia?
   A. dry, sticky mucous membranes
   B. headache
   C. muscle cramps
   D. thirst

5. Serum osmolality is a laboratory test that measures serum:
   A. concentration.
   B. pH.
   C. sodium levels.
   D. BUN.

6. Which of the following is *not* a complication of IV infusion therapy?
   A. filtration
   B. air embolus
   C. sepsis
   D. speed shock

CHAPTER 32

Links Between Nursing Science and Nursing Practice

■ BEHAVIORAL OBJECTIVES

After studying this chapter, you should be able to:

1. Discuss the importance of science as a way of knowing in nursing.

2. Describe nursing science both as a body of organized knowledge and as an approach to problem-solving.

3. List and describe the steps in the research process.

4. Discuss the evolution of theory in nursing.

5. Describe four major nursing models.

6. Describe the major nursing research methods.

7. Discuss the relationship between nursing science and practice and the ways in which nurse scientists and clinicians collaborate to conduct research.

■ KEY TERMS

applied science	design	null hypothesis
basic science	experimental method	operational definition
concept	explanatory theory	phenomenon
conceptual framework	holism	population
conceptual model	hypothesis	predictive theory
control	independent variable	qualitative research method
dependent variable	logical positivism	quantitative research method
descriptive theory	manipulation	randomization

random sample   research question   subjectivity
reliability   sample   theoretical framework
research   sampling error   theory
research hypothesis   science   validity
research problem   statistical method   variable

■ **REVIEW QUESTIONS**

1. Define science and explain why it is important for nurses to understand the nature of science as it relates to nursing.

2. List the ways a nurse can know if available nursing knowledge is adequate to guide nursing action, using Pierce's method of knowing.

3. Define:

    phenomenon

    concept

    theory

    validity

    reliability

4. Identify the levels of scientific theory.

5. Name the ten steps of the research process.

6. Differentiate among major research designs used in nursing.

7. Comment on the following: Quantitative research is superior to qualitative research.

8. Summarize four conceptual frameworks commonly used in nursing.

9. List six research methods used in nursing.

10. Describe the role of the nurse clinician in advancing nursing practice through nursing science.

■ ENRICHMENT ACTIVITIES

1. With a few of your classmates, discuss experiences with pain that each of you has had, describing your pain in terms of several dimensions such as nature, location, severity, frequency, duration, cause and alleviation, and so forth.   Based on your descriptions, can you devise a typology of pain? For example, were there instances of acute and chronic pain? Mild and severe pain? How would the setting in which the nurse works affect the typology of pain clients present? Consider a post-surgery unit. What types of pain might a nurse encounter? Would knowing the typology be of benefit in giving care? Why or why not?

2. The next time you are in the library, look at one or two journals that publish nursing research. Examples are: *Nursing Research; Journal of Advanced Nursing; Western Journal of Nursing Research;* and *Image: Journal of Nursing Scholarship.* How many of the articles would you classify as dealing with subjects related to the care of clients? What other topics are the subjects of nursing research? How many are related to professional issues or to nursing education? Which journal would you subscribe to in order to keep current?

3. While you are at the library, go to a computer terminal with a nursing database. Think of a nursing problem such as maintaining fluid intake in elderly clients or preventing pressure ulcers in clients who are immobile. Typing in related descriptors, how many research articles are you able to find on the topic in the last 5 years?

■ SELF-EXAMINATION QUESTIONS

1. The four concepts that bound the domain of nursing science are _____ _____, _____, and _____.

2. Theory development proceeds through three distinct levels: _____, _____, and _____.

3. List five rights of human subjects in research.

4. Match the research methods in column A with their definitions in column B.

		A		B
_____	(1)	clinical observation		a. an analysis drawn from one of a few subjects aimed at discovering the meaning of a phenomenon
_____	(2)	survey		
_____	(3)	phenomenological		b. studies various age groups or developmental stages at a single point in time to infer trends over time
_____	(4)	cross-sectional		
_____	(5)	retrospective		c. uses manipulation, control, and randomization to establish causal relationships
_____	(6)	longitudinal		
_____	(7)	experimental		

d. links subjects who presently demonstrate the phenomenon of interest to presumed causes occurring in the past

e. aims to describe the prevalence and distribution of a phenomenon in a population

f. examines events or phenomena over time in order to find time-ordered relationships

g. aims to define and describe a clinical phenomenon or situation

5. Match the nursing theorists in column A with their definitions of nursing in column B.

<u>A</u>

_____ (1) King

_____ (2) Orem

_____ (3) Roy

_____ (4) Rogers

<u>B</u>

a. a helping service focused on assisting a person to achieve self-care

b. a theoretical knowledge system prescribing analyses and actions when unusual stresses yield ineffective responses that threaten adaptation

c. a science directed at the study of unitary human development and an art aimed at promoting symphonic interaction between person and environment

d. an interpersonal process with the goal of helping individuals to maintain health

6. Ways in which a clinician can advance nursing practice by using nursing science include (choose as many answers as you think are correct):
    a. Read nursing journals in a specialty area.
    b. Write to your congressperson describing new nursing techniques discovered through research.
    c. Publish an interesting case study.
    d. Collect data from assigned clients.
    e. Volunteer to lecture to nursing students on a topic related to his or her expertise.
    f. Serve as a member of a research review committee.
    g. Join a professional association.

CHAPTER 33

Philosophy and Nursing Practice

■ **BEHAVIORAL OBJECTIVES**

After studying this chapter, you should be able to:

1. Describe how philosophic skills may be used in nursing practice.

2. Differentiate between empiricism and rationalism as descriptions of how knowledge is obtained.

3. Discuss the relevance of epistemology to nursing.

4. Explain the importance of metaphysical questions to nursing.

5. Define ethics.

6. Identify key assumptions of the mutual interaction model.

7. Differentiate between decision-making for the competent client and the incompetent client.

8. Identify values common to all theories of nursing.

9. Explain the difference between "providing care" and the caring approach to the client.

10. Use philosophy to explore personal reasons for choosing to become a nurse.

■ **KEY TERMS**

best interest standard	dualism	ethics
caring	empiricism	free will
determinism	epistemology	holism

metaphysics   philosophy   substituted judgment
Natural Law   rationalism   tacit assumption
philosophic argument

■ REVIEW QUESTIONS AND ACTIVITIES

1.   List the main types of philosophical methods.

2.   Distinguish between empiricism and rationalism.

3.   How does epistemology relate to the nursing process?

4.   Why is the metaphysical quest important in nursing?

5.   What branch of philosophy emphasizes whether actions are right or wrong?

6.   What are a few key assumptions of the mutual interaction model?

7. Using the case situations below, describe the differences between decision making for the competent client and incompetent client.

Case A
Mrs. Gowan, a 79-year-old with Alzheimer's disease (mid to late stage), is admitted to a local acute care facility from a nursing home. What evidence of substituted medical judgement will you look for in the medical record? Which standard of care can you use to reduce family conflict in making decisions?

Case B
Mrs. Coffee is a competent 73-year-old client with lung cancer whose prognosis is poor (less than 6 months to live). As the visiting nurse, how would you support her if she said, "I just don't want any more radiation treatment. I'd like to enjoy my family and their lives with the time I have left"?

8. Match the philosophic themes in column A with the correct theorists in column B.

A	B
_____ (1) free will and determination	a. Roy
_____ (2) mutual interaction model	b. Rogers
_____ (3) mind and body	c. Williamson
_____ (4) identity and change	d. Orem

9. Discuss the difference between caring for the client and just providing care.

10. State a personal value (e.g., love of technology, promoting independence in older adults) which you hold important in nursing practice. Write a sentence about how you use this value in your practice setting.

■ ENRICHMENT ACTIVITIES

1. Think about the experiences you had that convinced you to become a nurse. What was it that made nursing seem attractive? Can you identify the values that these experiences brought out, in yourself or in nursing, that provided the basis for your decision? For example, do you see yourself in the role of alleviating discomfort? Helping to cure illness? Working to help others adjust to their environments? Assisting people through life transitions? What clinical settings might offer the best opportunities for you to express such values? Can you connect your values with some of the philosophical issues discussed in the text, such as the mind-in-body dichotomy or free will?

2. Think about some of your first experiences in a clinical nursing setting where you were called upon to perform some aspects of nursing care. What were your feelings? Did you experience confusion? Can you identify some of the sources for your confusion, for example, the language or terminology used by other professionals or being asked to do something you had never done before? List as many sources as you can. What were some of the feelings you experienced in relation to not knowing immediately exactly what to do? How did you deal with this problem? Did you obtain information as a strategy? What sources of information did you use--asking others, reading, thinking, and problem solving? Were you able to cope in any of these situations simply by using your own powers of assessment and analysis? Which strategies did you rely on most often? What experiences helped you gain a sense of certainty in any of these situations? Is a sense of certainty important in nursing? In what kinds of situations? Might a sense of certainty ever be a hindrance in caregiving? In what situation?

3. Nursing situations can present many philosophical questions and ethical conflicts. It is important for nurses to know their own values on a variety of controversial issues as they pertain to health care. Think of an issue that might be particularly troubling to you, for example, keeping clients alive on life support systems when it is doubtful that their health will improve. What is your position? What is the source of your values on this issue? Does your belief put you into conflict with significant others or fellow students? Have your beliefs on this issue changed as a result of your education so far? If so, in what way?

4. With a friend, pick a controversial issue and take turns arguing for or against one side or the other on the issue. Make sure you each have an experience of arguing for a point of view that opposes your own beliefs. Does the experience of articulating opposing points of view change your own outlook at all?

■ SELF-EXAMINATION QUESTIONS

1. Match the terms in column A with the correct definitions from column B.

A	B
_____ (1) epistemology	a. perspective on the world, self, and people
_____ (2) value	b. assertion based on reasons
_____ (3) metaphysics	c. study of right and wrong
_____ (4) free will	d. a series of claims
_____ (5) philosophy	e. theory of knowledge
_____ (6) holism	f. choice

_____ (7) claim

_____ (8) ethics

_____ (9) philosophical argument

_____ (10) caring

g. belief about what is worthwhile

h. unified view of people

i. theory of reality

j. respect and regard for others

2. Fill in the blanks.

(1) Nursing research most often uses _____ epistemology.

(2) According to Descartes, true knowledge can only be gained by _____ .

(3) Roger's theory about change and development relates to the metaphysical issue of _____
_____ .

(4) Orem's theory of self-care agency raises the theme of_____.

(5) Roy's idea of the regulator and cognator is similar to the _____
issue in metaphysics.

(6) The view that people are a unity of mental, physical, and social aspects is known as _____.

(7) The nurse's respectful and considerate approach to others is known as a(n) _____
approach.

(8) Two key values of the mutual interaction or collaborative model of care are that clients _____
and _____ .

3. Match the types of clients in column A with the approaches in column B.

<u>A</u>

_____ (1) the alert, competent client

_____ (2) the incompetent client with a
living will

_____ (3) the incompetent client who has
left no advance directives

<u>B</u>

a. best interest standard

b. respect client's autonomous wishes

c. use substituted judgment

4. Place a T or F next to the statements below to indicate whether each is true or false.

_____ (1) Philosophy differentiates between good and bad reasons for entering nursing.
_____ (2) Philosophical methods can assist the nurse to provide higher quality care.
_____ (3) Epistemology is the study of right and wrong.
_____ (4) A hypothesis studies the causal relationship between two events.
_____ (5) Descartes believed that using experience is a good way to gain knowledge.
_____ (6) Nursing theories have some beliefs in common.
_____ (7) Nursing theories relate to philosophic issues.

_____ (8) The mutual interaction model states that the nurse's ideas are more important than those of the client.

_____ (9) A caring approach means that clients should always be given every available treatment.

_____ (10) Phenomenological research describes health care situations without using hypotheses.

5. According to Natural Law, people:
A. never change.
B. should attempt to make others as happy as possible.
C. have biological, rational, and social ends.
D. should eat natural food and develop a healthy life-style.

6. According to Carper, nursing knowledge has components of:
A. feeling, knowing, valuing, and thinking.
B. empathy, regard, and caring.
C. ethics, personal knowledge, aesthetics, and empirical information.
D. caring, healing, curing, and supporting.

CHAPTER 34

Values and Ethics in Nursing

■ **BEHAVIORAL OBJECTIVES**

After studying this chapter, you should be able to:

1. Define ethics.

2. Distinguish between an ethical dilemma and an ethical problem.

3. Identify personal values that have an impact on ethical decision-making.

4. Discuss seven steps in the process of acquiring values.

5. Identify professional values as expressed in codes of ethics and selected professional documents.

6. Identify professional values inherent in the mutual interaction model of nurse-client collaboration.

7. Identify eight general ethical principles that influence nursing practice.

8. Differentiate between the ethical theories of teleology and deontology.

9. Discuss caring as the basis of ethical behavior.

10. Identify several common ethical issues of nursing practice.

11. Resolve an ethical dilemma using a framework for justification.

12. Identify the ethical responsibilities of the professional nurse.

■ KEY TERMS

beneficence
client advocacy
code of ethics
confidentiality
deontology
deception
ethical dilemma
ethical principle
ethical problem

ethical theory
ethics
fidelity
justice
maxim
nonmaleficence
paternalism
personal value
prima facie duty

professional value
respect of autonomy
respect of person
teleology
theory of virtue
value
values clarification
value system
veracity

■ REVIEW QUESTIONS

1. Briefly define the term ethics.

2. Describe the difference between an ethical problem and an ethical dilemma.

3. Name the three action levels in the valuing process.

4. List the seven steps required in the valuing process.

5. State eight general ethical principles that influence nursing practice.

6. Describe the difference between teleology and deontology.

7. Match the professional values in column A with the correct documents in column B.

   <u>A</u>   <u>B</u>

   _____ (1) altruism   a.   CNA Code of Ethics

   _____ (2) accessible health care   b.   AACN Essential Values

   _____ (3) rights of nurses   c.   Social Policy Statement

   _____ (4) nondiscriminatory care   d.   ANA Code for Nurses

8. What four values are expressed in the mutual interaction model?

9. When can paternalism be justified?

10. Match the terms in column A with the correct definitions in column B.

    <u>A</u>   <u>B</u>

    _____ (1) excellence   a.   standing up for clients

    _____ (2) thinking   b.   sense of self as moral agent

    _____ (3) holism   c.   respecting persons as unified beings

    _____ (4) integrity   d.   fidelity in upholding professional standards

    _____ (5) collaboration   e.   demonstrating critical reasoning

    _____ (6) advocacy   f.   being clinically competent

    _____ (7) loyalty   g.   being committed to mutual interaction

■ ENRICHMENT ACTIVITIES

1. *Personal values clarification exercise*: List the things you value.   Try to list 15 to 20 things. Pick the 10 things you value most from your list and number them from 1 (most important) to 10. On a separate page make two columns. In the left column list all of your activities from yesterday. If yesterday was a Sunday, list all of your activities for the entire weekend. In the right column list the value represented in each of the activities. For example:

Activity	Value
• Soda break with friend	• Friendship or relaxation
• Library work	• Gaining knowledge, or professional goal, or good grades

    Return to your original list of the 10 things you value most and compare it with the values listed on the activity page. Talk with a friend about what you discovered about yourself in this exercise.

2. As you think of your basic values, try to identify clinical situations in which you believe you would have difficulty in providing nursing care. Some examples of clinical situations in which nurses sometimes face conflicts in values are abortion, the right to die, withholding food and water, and genetic testing to determine fetal handicaps. Do you believe that you could justify not providing care in any specific nursing situation? Discuss with friends the situation in which there would be no exception for you, that is, the situation in which you would absolutely not participate, regardless of the consequences.

3. Join with one or two friends in this values exercise. Individually read the letters to the editor in one local newspaper and one professional journal. Jot down the value or values reflected in each letter. Consider your own perspective on the topics. What values are represented in your inclinations to action or inaction? Discuss reactions with your friends, listening carefully to the others' perspectives. Discuss what topics or issues would motivate each of you to write a letter to the editor. What values are presented in such action?

■ SELF-EXAMINATION QUESTIONS

1. Give a brief example of an ethical dilemma.

2. List five values that are expressed publicly by the nursing profession.

3. Match the ethical principles in column A with the best definition in column B.

           <u>A</u>   <u>B</u>

_____ (1) beneficence   a.   telling the truth

_____ (2) respect of person   b.   keeping promises

_____ (3) fidelity   c.   doing good for another

_____ (4) confidentiality   d.   allowing client self-determination

_____ (5) nonmaleficence   e.   preventing harm

_____ (6) veracity   f.   maintaining privacy

_____ (7) respect of autonomy   g.   treating others with regard and concern

_____ (8) justice   h.   the fair distribution of goods and services

4. The primary question of the teleologist is:
    A. What is my duty?
    B. What is God's law?
    C. What rights are being violated?
    D. What will produce good consequences?

5. The primary question of the deontologist is:
    A. What is my duty?
    B. What is God's law?
    C. What rights are being violated?
    D. What will produce good consequences?

6. State the four criteria of autonomy.

7. List the three criteria used to justify paternalistic action.

8. Justification of action from an ethical perspective always includes an appeal to _____.

CHAPTER 35

Health Care Delivery

- ## BEHAVIORAL OBJECTIVES

After studying this chapter, you should be able to:

1. Name at least three health-related functions carried out by the federal, state, and local governments.

2. Compare and contrast fee-for-service, capitation, and fee-for-diagnosis methods of health care payment.

3. Describe the third-party payment system currently used in the United States.

4. Define what is meant by a health maintenance organization.

5. Briefly discuss the original intent of the Medicare program and discuss one major factor that has altered the implementation of this program.

6. Discuss the original intent of the Medicaid program.

7. Define Medicare's prospective payment system and the diagnostic related group (DRG).

8. Discuss attempts by insurance companies, employers, community health care services, health care providers, and the federal government to reduce health care costs.

9. Discuss the effects of changing population demographics for the health care system.

10. Discuss factors that can encourage the client to become an active health care consumer.

11. Identify and explain two major challenges facing the nurse in promoting cost-conscious health care.

12. Identify two implications for the nursing profession resulting from the lack of third-party reimbursement for nursing services.

■ **KEY TERMS**

accreditation
ambulatory care
capitation
case managers
certification
employee medical benefits
fee-for-diagnosis
fee-for-service

health maintenance organization
home care
hospice care
managed care
Medicaid
Medicare
peer review
peer review organization

primary care
prospective payment system
quality of care
secondary care
self-monitoring review system
tertiary care
utilization review

■ **REVIEW QUESTIONS**

1. Why is it important for nurses to have an understanding of the organizational structure of government and the roles played by the government in facilitating and providing health care services?

2. List the ways that federal, state, and local governments, respectively, carry out at least one health-related function.

3. Define:

    accreditation

    utilization review

    health maintenance organization

    hospice care

    managed care

4. Identify three types of billing for health care services.

5. Name the main sources of payment for care.

6. Differentiate between Medicare and Medicaid.

7. Summarize four of the circumstances that have led to the present problems in health care.

8. List six cost-control strategies the government has used to stem the rising costs of health care.

9. What activities have community health centers developed to maximize individual wellness?

10. Describe the key elements of nursing's agenda for health care reform.

■ ENRICHMENT ACTIVITIES

1. Identify four different types of health care providers in your community (specific practioners, clinics, agencies, institutions) who exemplify the values of wellness, disease prevention, and health promotion in health care delivery. State the rationale for your choices and document your basis for choosing them. Did you use ads, refer to lists of services, check credentials, infer from the name of the clinic or agency, speak to their providers? Compare your list with those of fellow students who live in the same and in different areas.

2. Talk to several fellow students about health care providers they have used. Consider, for example, podiatrists, pharmacists, chiropractors, optometrists, orthodontists, family dentists, pediatricians, physical therapists, and nutritionists. Compare ideas, based on your own experience, about what these providers do--what the focus of their practice is and what types of services they provide. Specifically, what type of health care problems could each treat?

3. Look in the local Yellow Pages for ads for health care providers. What types are listed? What services do they render based on the ad copy? Do the ads suggest limitations to the provider's practice? Based on the ads, how would you evaluate the provider's ideas of what is important to the consumer?

4. Ask several fellow students whether they have health insurance. If so, what type is it, what services are covered, and which services are not covered? Discuss experiences in making claims. What was involved? Who processed the claim? How much of the bill did the insurance cover? Did they experience difficulties in the claim process? How did they handle them?

5. Follow the local news in your city's major newspaper for two weeks. What types of health care issues are covered? What city and county agencies are mentioned? Based on the articles you find, what would you say are the most important health issues in your area?

■ **SELF-EXAMINATION QUESTIONS**

1. Match the health care functions in column A with the levels of government engaging in them in column B.

<u>A</u>   <u>B</u>

_____ (1) collect statistics on diseases   a. federal

_____ (2) provide financial assistance to educational institutions   b. state

    c. local

_____ (3) provide financial assistance to help citizens over the age 65 meet medical expenses

_____ (4) administer a self-supporting retirement plan for citizens

_____ (5) license health care providers

_____ (6) license health care facilities

_____ (7) manage school health programs

2. True or false:

_____ Clients treated in an emergency treatment center usually require intense medical supervision.

_____ Government tax money is not available to meet the cost of home health care.

_____ Hospice care may include the services of thanatology specialists, providers who have studied the dying process.

3. True or false:

_____ A peer review organization (PRO) is an organization composed of professionals that provides a retrospective review of the care provided by all providers in a facility.

_____   The research requirements of the Food and Drug Administration assure the consumer that the manufacturer has thoroughly investigated the effectiveness of its foods, drugs, or cosmetics.

_____   HSAs are one of the most effective local agencies for ensuring against duplication of health care facilities.

4. Private-sector regulation is important in controlling the quality of health care.   Which of the following organizations are involved in certifying (formally recognizing an individual's competence) in nursing?
   A. National Association of the American College of Obstetricians and Gynecologists
   B. American Nurses' Association
   C. National League for Nursing
   D. Joint Commission on the Accreditation of Healthcare Organizations

5. Match the types of payment system in column A with the correct descriptions in column B.

	<u>A</u>		<u>B</u>
_____	(1) fee for service	a.	facility is given a fixed dollar amount based on the client's age and diagnosis before services are provided
_____	(2) capitation		
_____	(3) fee for diagnosis	b.	consumer pays for each health service as it is provided
		c.	a set fee is paid to cover all health services provided in a given period

6. All of the following are examples of government health plans *except:*
   A. voluntary insurance.
   B. Medicare.
   C. Medicaid.
   D. veterans' benefits.

CHAPTER 36

Economics in Health Care and Nursing

■ **BEHAVIORAL OBJECTIVES**

After studying this chapter, you should be able to:

1. Define economics.

2. State the importance of economics in health care and describe its contribution to the functioning of the health care system.

3. Explain how resources are allocated within the economy and within the health care system.

4. Discuss the concepts of efficiency and effectiveness in producing health care services.

5. List the decisions that must be made by an economic system.

6. Describe the conflict that arises between individuals and society in the use of health care services.

7. State the fundamental conditions for a competitive market.

8. List factors that affect the demand for health care services.

9. List factors that affect the supply of health care services.

10. List the distinctive economic characteristics of the US health care system and discuss their implications.

11. Identify several differences between the way economics works in the health care system and in most other industries.

12. Define cost-benefit analysis and cost-effectiveness analysis and state their uses in health care.

13. State the relevance of economics to nursing and nurses.

14. Describe how nurses can use economics in collaborating with clients in their care.

■ **KEY TERMS**

accountability   economies of scale   price elasticity
capitalism   effectiveness   productivity
capitation   efficiency   rational economic behavior
case management   managed care   socialism
derived demand   monopoly power   utility
economic resources   monopsony power   utilization management
economics   multi-institutional systems

■ **REVIEW QUESTIONS**

1. Define economics and explain why it is important for nurses to understand the importance of economics in health care.

2. Define:

    efficiency

    productivity

    effectiveness

    economic resources

    accountability

3. Identify two types of economic systems.

4. What are the basic components of the market system?

5. List the main characteristics of a competitive market.

6. How do demand and supply in the market work together?

7. List the characteristics of the health care industry that interfere with market self-correction.

8. List six levels of economic decision making within the health care industry.

9. List six levels of economic decision making for nurses in the health care industry.

10. Describe how individual nurses make economic decisions about their priorities for providing direct client care.

■ ENRICHMENT ACTIVITIES

1.   Look around the room you are in. Focus on one item. Consider that item as a product. What raw materials were involved in its production? From what parts of the world did these materials come? How was the item made? How many different suppliers contributed materials? What types of workers were necessary to assemble the item? Think about similar items you have seen and the different models and colors in which the item is available. What is the approximate price range for the product? Why do you suppose the price varies from model to model?

2.   The next time you go to the drug store, look at the various health care products on the shelves. Pick one, for instance bandages or gauze dressings. Ask yourself the questions in activity 1. Look at the prices of the competing brands. What might account for the differences in price? What economic considerations should be made in choosing one product over the others?

3.   For one week, clip newspaper articles about specific economic decisions made at different levels of the decision-making pyramid. Who is involved in the decisions? Were the issues involved specific to a firm, to an individual, to a group, to society as a whole? What kinds of decisions were made about health care? What decision-making level was involved? Who was involved in the decision making? What were their roles?

■ SELF-EXAMINATION QUESTIONS

1.   What decisions must any economic system make?

2.   What unique characteristics does the health care system possess?

3.   What are the steps involved in cost-benefit analysis?

4.   What determines the demand for health care?

5.   Why is an understanding of economics important to the practice of nursing?

CHAPTER 37

Health Care as a Transaction

■ **BEHAVIORAL OBJECTIVES**

After studying this chapter, you should be able to:

1. Define the transaction concept as it pertains to health care.

2. Summarize several factors that influence the delivery and cost of health care, and list the major barriers to health care access in the United States.

3. Describe the policy alternatives for achieving the goal of universal access to health care.

4. Describe four moral arguments for a right to health care.

5. Define consumerism, list several rights and obligations of consumers, and describe the place of consumerism in health care transactions.

6. List obstacles to consumer decision making in health care and discuss ways nurses can help clients to become successful consumers.

7. State the difference between a "disease paradigm" and an "illness paradigm" for viewing sickness and discuss the relevance of the transactional approach to provider-client relationships.

8. Define collaboration.

9. List the assumptions and describe the phases of the mutual interaction model of client care.

10. Discuss what is meant by a client contract and discuss its role in collaboration.

11. List client- and nurse-related variables influencing the use of the mutual interaction model.

12. State the relationship between mutual-interaction, adherence, and caring.

13. Discuss the role of negotiation in collaboration, and define what is meant by consensus-building.

14. State several approaches to clients that promote principled negotiation.

■ **KEY TERMS**

adherence	individualism	power resource
agenda decisions	influence	principled negotiation
collaboration	leadership	program decisions
collaborative decision-making	management	shared governance
consensus building	management by objectives	transaction
consumerism	mutual interaction	transformational leadership
control	operational control decisions	

■ **REVIEW QUESTIONS**

1. Discuss what is meant by health care as an economic transaction.

2. Define:

consumerism

management by objectives

mutual interaction

shared governance

transformational leadership

collaboration

3. Identify problems in achieving distributive justice in health care.

4. What are some alternatives to the current health care system?

5. Name the main aspects of the Consumer Bill of Rights.

6. Discuss the phases in the mutual interaction model.

7. List the guidelines for negotiating and consensus building.

8. List the management functions of nurse managers in health care agencies.

9. Discuss Maslow's, McClelland's and Hertzberg's theories of motivation.

10. Describe the four fundamental characteristics of leadership.

■ ENRICHMENT ACTIVITIES

1.   Think about the last time you went to a physician. What were the reasons you sought care? Did you also see a nurse? Was the interaction with the health care providers you saw collaborative? In what way? What would you have done to make it more collaborative?

2.   Considering the same experience, what did you do in your role as health care consumer? Can you describe behavior oriented toward gaining information or asserting yourself in decision making that is consistent with the consumer role? Talk to some friends about their use of the consumer role in seeking health care. How did they find the providers they use? What were the sources of their information about providers? Have any of them ever sought a second opinion about a medical diagnosis or treatment recommendation? How might a nurse help clients to understand the importance of such behavior?

3.   The next time you go to a clinical setting, listen closely to the providers as they talk with each other and talk with clients. Listen for examples of the use of paternalistic and collaborative language. Are there some providers who seem to assume more of a partnership role than others as evidenced in their language? Discuss your findings with a few fellow students and compare observations.

4.   With a fellow student, role-play a client care situation in which principled negotiation might be used, with one of you assuming the client role and the other the nurse role. Consider, for example, the client who declines to ambulate following surgery, but who shows signs of pulmonary congestion. The person playing the client role can invent the reasons for declining; the person playing the nurse's role takes on the task of working toward a negotiated consensus with the client. After you reach a compromise or an impasse, analyze the nurse's approaches for their effectiveness in the situation. Was the focus on interest rather than positions? Were the decision criteria objective?

5.   Again with a fellow student, discuss the behavior of several nurses you both are familiar with as to whether it constitutes characteristics of either good management or leadership. Does the unit manager of the unit to which you are assigned also act as a leader? Describe the behavior that supports your position.

■ SELF-EXAMINATION QUESTIONS

1.   Consumerism refers to:
      A. resistance to provider influence.
      B. promotion of consumer interests.
      C. skepticism regarding provider motives.
      D. advocating informed consent.

2.   List four historical influences on consumerism in health care.

3.   Identify three areas in which health care consumers have difficulty and are likely to require assistance.

4. Which of the following moral arguments provides the *weakest* position for establishing health care as a right?
    A. utilitarianism
    B. egalitarianism
    C. libertarianism
    D. contractarianism

5. Which of the following was *not* a historical influence on the emerging emphasis of collaboration in health care?
    A. consumerism
    B. informed consent movement
    C. civil rights movement
    D. emergence of managed care

6. Which of the following is true of the exploratory phase of the mutual interaction model?
    A. an initial period of contact between client and nurse
    B. a phase in which issues are clarified and perceptions shared
    C. a period in which desired outcomes are defined
    D. a phase in which strategies are explored and selected

7. Why is it important to separate one's positions from one's interests under principled negotiation?

8. List several roles that the manager of a nursing unit might play.

■ CHAPTER 1

Review Questions

1. A. Respect the rights of others.
    B. Provide the best care that current knowledge and technology offers.
    C. Recognize clients' right to informed consent.
    D. Accept the need for cost-effective practice. (Page 11)

2. A. More men and minorities are entering nursing.
    B. Increasing numbers of nurses are seeking master's degrees with a focus on advanced clinical practice.
    (Pages 7-8)

3. Licensure, certification, accreditation (Page 16)

4. (1) b, (2) d, (3) a, (4) c (Page 6)

5.
Caring	Compassion	Concern
Coping behaviors	Empathy	Enabling
Facilitating	Interest	Involvement
Health consultative acts	Health instruction acts	Health maintenance acts
Helping behaviors	Love	Nurturance
Protective behaviors	Restorative behaviors	Sharing
Stimulating behaviors	Stress alleviation	Succorance
Support	Surveillance	Tenderness (Page 5)
Touching	Trust	

6. Humanistic altruistic system of values
    Faith-hope
    Sensitivity to self and others
    Helping-trusting human care relationship
    Expressing positive and negative feelings
    Creative problem-solving caring process
    Transpersonal teaching-learning
    Supportive, protective, and/or corrective mental, physical, societal, and spiritual environment
    Human needs assistance
    Existential-phenomenological-spiritual forces (Page 5)

7. Prescribed program of advanced education, concern with matters of significance, continuing intellectual pursuits, self-regulation of entry and practice within the profession (Page 5)

8. (1) c, (2) d, (3) b, (4) a (Page 20)

9. Case nursing--One nurse gives total care to one or more clients for an entire shift.
    Functional nursing--Work assignments are organized according to tasks, rather than total care to a client.
    Team nursing--Care planning and work assignments are collaboratively carried out by the team leader (RN), and team members (RNs, LVNs, nurse's aides).

Primary nursing--Primary nurse (RN) assumes responsibility for care planning and around-the-clock coordination of care for one or more clients during their entire hospital stay, as well as providing care when on duty. Associate nurses (RNs) provide care when primary nurse is not on duty. (Page 21)

10. Hospitals, communities, nursing homes, private duty, education (Page 17)

Self-Examination Questions

1. The diagnosis and treatment of human responses to actual or potential health problems

2. (1) c, (2) a, (3) d, (4) f, (5) b, (6) e

3. Mutual understanding, mutual trust, mutual control, and mutual responsibility

4. Schools, clinics, nursing homes, and workplace

5. Individual; program

6. Diploma, associate degree, baccalaureate, and master's degree (MN or MSN) or nurse doctorate (ND)

■ CHAPTER 2

Review Questions

1. Possible answers to this question include: intellectual pursuit of a body of knowledge; practice guided by a body of theory, a community of shared values; a code of ethics; focus on matters of human urgency and significance; autonomy, control, and accountability in practice. (Pages 25-26)

2. (1) e, (2) a, (3) f, (4) b, (5) d, (6) c (Pages 30-31)

3. Possible answers include: role transition from student to nurse; changing practice roles from gereralist to specialist; changing functional roles from teacher to administrator to researcher; reconciling high-tech with high-touch practice issues. (Pages 40-41)

4. (1) g, (2) c, (3) a, (4) e, (5) d, (6) h, (7) b, (8) f (Pages 35-36)

5. Rights: regulate entry into nursing practice; review and sanction peers; receive fair compensation for service; provide direct service to clients for direct reimbursement; show pride in nursing as a profession. (Page 44)
   Responsibilities: address crucial current issues; model a professional image; educate consumers; be active in professional organizations; collaborate with other providers to influence health policy (Page 43)

6. Changing economics. (Rapidly rising health care costs are forcing consumers to pay more out of their own pockets as recipients of health care.)
   Changing consumers. (Consumers are more informed, more assertive, and more participative about their health and health care choices.)
   Sophisticated technology, which keeps alive individuals at both ends of the life span. (This is very costly and requires long-term care settings. Nursing can influence the organization and delivery of services in these settings.)
   Limited access to health care services. (A growing segment of the population, mostly poor, has no health insurance coverage. An increasing part of the work force also has limited or no health insurance.

These groups are a high-risk and vulnerable population that will increase demands on nursing to provide cost-effective alternatives to traditional medical models for health care.)

Increasing number of elderly. (This will require a fuller involvement of nurses in the development of a range of services that improve the quality of life and promote healthy aging.) (Pages 44-45)

7. A job is a series of routine, frequently repetitive tasks, often undertaken for the sole purpose of receiving monetary compensation. Individuals who perceive their work as a job only often lack long-range goals or commitment to an institution or its clients.

   On the other hand, a profession is a career. Professional nurses plan a career, develop long-range goals, move through a series of nursing positions, and make a contribution to the profession. Completion of their career goals leads to personal recognition and rewards other than monetary compensation. (Page 42)

8. Possible answers to this question include: formation of coalitions and alliances with consumers; greater involvement in professional organizations and in health care policy development; assuming administrative control of skilled nursing facilities and home health care services; and reforming health care systems and nursing practice to ensure high quality health care services, especially for the poor and the elderly. (Page 46)

9. Autonomy is the freedom to choose one's actions. Professional autonomy in nursing refers to self-directed clinical practice. Steps toward this long-range goal in nursing include shared governance and participative management structures in place in some health care organizations.

   Control implies direction or regulation over someone or something. For professional nursing this means the authority to control the practice of nursing by determining the roles, functions, and responsibilities of its members.

   Accountability is taking responsibility for one's actions. In nursing this means that nurses are directly responsible to their clients for the quality of nursing care provided. (Page 27)

10. The feminist movement has had both positive and negative effects on the profession of nursing. On the positive side the women's movement has raised the consciousness of the public about how society views women, the socialization of women, equal opportunities and pay, and the right to be free from sexual harassment. On the negative side it raised barriers to nursing during the late 1960's and early 1970's by discouraging bright young women from entering occupations such as nursing and teaching and encouraging them instead to enter male-dominated fields such as engineering, business, law, and medicine. More recently, feminism has been concerned with such issues as gaining social acceptance and placing value on such qualities as caring and nurturing. (Pages 37-38)

Self-Examination Questions

1. A. Body of knowledge: increases in nursing research
    B. Body of theory: beginning nursing theories
    C. Attention to matters of human concern and urgency: focus on caring for people; emphasis on health care promotion and prevention
    D. Code of ethics: published Code for Nurses by ANA

2. C

3. (1) c, (2) a, (3) b, (4) e, (5) d

4. Professional trend: The introduction of the concept of nursing diagnosis in the 1950s was a significant contribution to the development of nursing as a science.

    Socio-political trend: Wars, and the shortages of trained personnel they create, have given considerable socio-political impetus to the development of nursing service and nursing education. After World War II, serious nursing shortages led to a proliferation of paraprofessional hospital personnel and an end to nursing's exclusive role in the care of the sick. The Korean War motivated the development of a system of technical education in nursing.

5.   (1) b,   (2) e,   (3) a,   (4) d,   (5) c

6.   Sexism, paternalism, rapid changes in technology, conflicting social expectations, devalued feminine image

■ **CHAPTER 3**

Review Questions

1.   Constitutional law, statutory law, common law, administrative regulation. (Page 52)

2.   (1) d,   (2) c,   (3) a,   (4) b   (Pages 52-53)

3.   Answers to this questions include: fraud and deceit, incompetence, criminal activity, unethical practice, drug or alcohol abuse, negligence, and violation of the Nurse Practice Act.   (Page 60)

4.   A Nurse Practice Act includes: a definition of nursing; requirements for licensure (initial and renewal); exceptions to the practice act; options that apply in special circumstances; actions or conditions that can cause loss or limitation of a license; and administrative structure that implements and administers the practice act. (Page 54)

5.   A.   The defendant had a legally recognized duty to provide health care to the client.
      B.   The defendant breached this duty by providing substandard care.
      C.   Physical and mental damages to the plaintiff resulted.
      D.   The direct cause of these damages was the breach of care by the defendant.   (Page 64)

6.   True. Limitations on advanced medical practice are primarily from peer pressure. Although some requirements of insurance companies, accreditation standards, and laws of licensure specify certification for advanced practice in medicine, medical practice acts have yet to make this distinction.   (Page 57)

7.   Resources available to nurses for advice regarding legal and/or ethical problems include but are not limited to: practice acts for nursing and other professions; hospital and other health facility licensing laws; public health, safety, insurance, and education codes; and laws relating to the rights of clients.   (Page 65)

8.   Examples of client rights include: informed consent; the right to refuse treatment; the right to die/right to life; and access to care.   (Pages 66-71)

9.   Licensure is a device for the protection of the public good. It is a state, not federal, function. Licensure grants an individual the right to provide certain professional services. Licenses may be weak or absolute. Original registration acts that covered nursing practice were weak or limited. Medical practice acts are examples of very strong acts. Nurse practice acts continue to grow stronger, especially in the area of advanced practice, but are not yet as strong as medical practice acts. (Page 53)

10.   Possible answers include: treating clients and families with respect and honesty; documenting all nursing care and clients' responses to nursing care clearly, completely, and concisely; delegating client care; adhering to agency policies and procedures; knowing state's Nurse Practice Act; and attending continuing education programs.   (Page 63)

Self-Examination Questions

1. Protecting the public, defining scope of practice, defining education requirements, limiting rights to perform certain functions

2. Durable power of attorney

3. D

4. Good samaritan law

5. Negligence, incompetence

6. C

■ CHAPTER 4

Review Questions

1. A. Issue or problem development (for example, the need for national health insurance)
    B. Consensus-building about the issue by a group of concerned individuals (for example, farmers and health care activists improved the nutrition of pregnant women, infants, and children through the WIC program)
    C. Setting an agenda so the policy receives sufficient attention (for example, White House Conference on Aging)
    D. Converting policy into laws through the legislative process (for example, amending the Nurse Practice Acts in individual states)   (Pages 77-78)

2. Political involvement is an important part of every nurse's professional role. Individual nurses can become involved in health care issues at the local, state, or national levels. A good way to begin is to join the lobbying efforts of a professional organization. Prescription-writing privileges for nurses in the advanced practice role is an example of an issue that has been successfully lobbied and enacted into law in some states by professional organizations   (ANA and the Nurse Practitioner Association). (Pages 90-91)

3. A. Suggesting or initiating legislation
    B. Testifying before legislative committees
    C. Belonging to professional organizations
    D. Shaping public opinion.
    E. Establishing lobbying relationships (Pages 92-93)

4. A. Letters to legislators
    B. Telephone calls to legislators
    C. Personal visits to legislators
    D. Attending public hearings
    E. Testifying at public hearings
    F. Maintaining the relationship through follow-up letters and/or meetings (Pages 94-95)

5. Do prepare ahead, introduce yourself, share a personal point of reference, and let them know whom you are representing; express appreciation for past services or support. Don't lie, exaggerate, or misrepresent yourself; focus your energy on officials who have already publicly stated their positions; lose your temper or use harsh or profane words. (Page 94)

6. Federal: allocation of money for programs such as Medicare
    State: eligibility for licensure, eligibility for Medicaid
    County: policy decisions regarding public health nursing services, school health regulations, and water and
        pollution control
    Municipal: health insurance for city or town employees control of communicable disease, and surveillance of
        restaurants and schools for compliance with Board of Health requirements (Pages 76-77)

7. Individuals or groups use politics, the art or science of government, as power to guide or influence policy
    decisions. Policy identifies goals and purposes and defines priorities that influence the government's decisions
    about how to solve problems. Laws and regulations that specifically define the government's course of action
    are then enacted at federal, state, and municipal levels. (Page 76)

8. Decisions are made in our political system by voting. Our elected officials make allocation decisions, for
    example, by voting. Citizens can determine the outcome of policies by influencing officials who do the lobbying
    or voting. (Pages 84-85)

9. A. Legitimate power, or the power inherent in a position. For example, a head nurse can make changes in
        the schedules of nursing staff.
    B. Reward power, or the ability to grant favors or benefits. For example, a politician can appoint an
        individual who supported his campaign to a government position.
    C. Coercive power, or the use of punishment. For example, an elected official can dismiss an individual
        appointed by a previous administration.
    D. Expert power, which is derived from knowledge and information.
    E. Referent power, by which the force of an individual's or organization's reputation influences decisions.
        For example, noted nursing scholars or the ANA can influence nursing procedures.
    F. Personal power is exerted through the force of an individual's personality.
    G. Collective power is exerted through collective movements and social groups. Civil rights and the women's
        movement are examples. (Pages 88-89)

10. A. Political action committees (groups of individuals who work to elect candidates who will support the policy
        interests of the group once elected)
    B. Campaign contributions
    C. Grass-roots participation such as stuffing envelopes, answering telephones, distributing leaflets, and
        soliciting support for candidates (Page 86)

Self-Examination Questions

1. Policy formation, legislative process, policy implementation, and policy evaluation

2. General; specific

3. True

4. Letters, telegrams, mailgrams, telephone calls, personal visits, oral testimony, and written testimony

5. False

6. False

■ CHAPTER 5

Review Questions

1. It is important for nurses to have clear definitions of these terms because health beliefs influence health practices, and a nurse's definitions will influence the scope of nursing practice. (Page 103)

2. Genetic identity, environment, social and cultural factors, individual behavior (Page 106)

3. Nurses act as resources, educators, role models, and motivators. (Page 107)

4. Nurses promote health through role-modeling in many ways; for example, by not smoking, by avoiding sunburn, and by maintaining a nutritious diet. (Page 107)

5. Strengths: health as a continuum; health and illness not fixed but always changing
   Limitation: does not account for moving toward greater health in one area, while at the same time moving toward lesser health in other areas (Page 111)

6. (1) b, (2) c, (3) a, (4) d   (Page 113)

7. Cardiovascular disease--weight loss programs; cancer of the skin--education about excessive sunning; accidents--driving instruction for teenagers; chronic obstructive lung disease--stop smoking programs; pneumonia --immunization for high-risk groups (Page 112)

8. Primary prevention--teaching, role-modeling
   Secondary prevention--screening
   Tertiary prevention--teaching a client who smokes how to stop (Page 113)

9. Client education: Provide information regarding relationship of weight to hypertension. (Page 112)

10. The prevalence of hypertension in black populations, the consequences for her children, and personal responsibility (Page 114)

Self-Examination Questions

1. C

2. (1) b, (2) d, (3) a, (4) c

3. False

4. Act as a resource, an educator, a role model, and a motivator

5. False

6. Determine whether the decision is an informed decision, based on correct and complete information about the benefits of the change(s) and the risks of continuing current behavior.

■ **CHAPTER 6**

Review Questions

1.   Change in individuals is defined as a continuous process in which differences in ways of being or functioning occur relative to past ways of functioning. (Page 122)

2.   The change process consists of unfreezing, moving, and refreezing. Applied to smoking: Unfreezing--assess health; learn about problems related to smoking and benefits of not smoking; decide to stop smoking. Moving --stop smoking; join a support group; change behaviors surrounding smoking. Refreezing--maintain new behavior for one year. (Page 122)

3.   Does Mr. Edward view the change as threatening? Is his reaction healthy? How does the change affect his interaction with his family and his ability to function? (Page 126)

4.   Factors that enable or impede one's ability to deal with stress include: (A) mediating factors: number of stressors, duration of event, intensity of the event, availability of social and financial resources; (B) the ability to resist stress: genetics, lifestyle, sense of humor, self-confidence, security, adequate resources. (Pages 136- 140)

5.   Mr. James' stress is related to his job and to his personal life. He has described physical and emotional signs of stress (can't sleep, overeats, is tired and agitated, does not care about his clothes). His ability to adapt to stress seems to be exhausted, and without help his physical health will deteriorate. (Page 139)

6.   The nurse should help Mr. James cope by helping him to determine his usual coping strategies and what is working for him. Discuss the major stressors and the daily hassles in his life, and monitor physiological signs of stress. Assess support systems, and encourage collaboration. (Page 141)

7.   Review the recent stress in Mrs. Power's life, monitor physiological parameters, assess support systems, encourage collaboration, and teach coping mechanisms. (Page 141)

8.   Mrs. Powers is in an actual crisis situation and her usual coping mechanisms are failing. Her resources are overwhelmed. The problem has no end, and she cannot envision a way out. The family does not know what to do. (Page 140)

9.   The stresses of nursing include: working conditions; work hours; shortages of nurses; working with the needy; pressure to keep up with information; constraints of time and resources; and working with clients whose lives are at stake. (Page 142)

10. Stress management techniques for nurses include: take stock of yourself; identify your strengths and weaknesses; take care of yourself; take stock of your stressors; cultivate coping measures; develop a support network; take control of your work situation; manage your time effectively; be wary of making mistakes; avoid emotional overinvolvement; acknowledge the meaning of caring. (Page 143)

Self-Examination Questions

1.   Autonomic nervous system; endocrine system

2.   (1) a, (2) b, (3) a, (4) a

3.   D

4. C

5. D

6. D

7. A

■ **CHAPTER 7**

Review Questions

1. Community health is a composite of the health status of individuals, families, and groups within the population and the ability of the group to carry out certain necessary functions. In this text, the terms community health and public health are interchangeable. It is important for nurses to understand community health because nurses play an important role in maintaining and improving the health of the community. Nurses are actively involved in health promotion and the prevention of community health problems, an endeavor that requires specific knowledge of the factors that affect health in the community. (Pages 156-157)

2. The two major sectors of the health care delivery system in the United States are: (1) The acute care sector, which refers to health professionals in hospitals, clinics, and other settings who treat people who become ill. This sector emphasizes curing disease and restoring health. The focus is on the individual, although assistance is given to the family. (2) The community health sector encompasses the health professionals who keep people from becoming ill. They work in various settings, such as schools, homes, clinics of various types, and hospitals. The community health sector emphasizes health promotion and illness prevention rather than cure of illness. The primary focus of the community health sector is on the total population not the health of the individual. Community health provides services to individuals and families but does so because such services enhance the health of the group. (Page 157)

3. The five categories are health education, health appraisal, life-style modification, providing a healthy environment, and developing coping skills. (Page 157)

4. Strategies for health promotion include teaching about infant immunizations, handwashing in caring for the baby, adequate nutrition and rest for the mother and baby, signs of fever and infection, when to call the health care center, safety, and protection from poisons. (Page 170)

5. Epidemiology is the study of factors that affect the occurrence of disease. By understanding the principles of epidemiology, health care professionals can take an intelligent approach to both disease prevention and health promotion. The epidemiological triad examines health problems in three categories: Agent factors, host factors, and environmental factors. By understanding each component of a disease, nurses can analyze, understand and predict patterns of disease and devise strategies for disease control (Page 160)

6. According to Pender, health promotion is not disease- or health-problem specific. It seeks to expand the positive potential for health. Disease prevention focuses on threats to health and the need to protect people in the community. (Pages 176-177)

7. Strategies to explore include: (a) primary prevention: education to stop smoking, stress reduction, exercise program, weight reduction, coping skills; (b) secondary prevention: early diagnosis of cardiac problems, watching blood pressure, weight control, cholesterol levels. (Page 173)

8. Risk factors for diabetes mellitus include obesity and genetic predisposition. Prevention strategies include: Primary: weight reduction, cessation of smoking; Secondary: Monitor urine and blood sugar, treat with insulin or oral hypoglycemics; Tertiary: prevent complications and general deterioration caused by disease. (Page 175)

9. Community health nursing includes: (a) client-oriented roles (health educator, counselor, referral resource, liaison, advocate, role model, direct care provider, (b) delivery-oriented roles, (coordinator, collaborator, discharge planner, supervisor) (c) community-oriented roles (case finder, community assessor, program planner, evaluator) and (d) researcher and research user. (Pages 180-184)

10. Began in England--Florence Nightingale; Lillian Wald, first organized nursing efforts at Henry Street Settlement; 1898, Los Angeles became first municipality to employ community health nurses; Met Life Insurance in 1909 hired nurses for home nursing services; 1923, Community Health Nursing reinforced by Goldmark Report; 1963, Neighborhood Health Center Act provided federal assistance to community health centers. (Page 179)

Self-Examination Questions

1. (1) b, (2) a, (3) d, (4) f, (5) c

2. B

3. Agent factors, host factors, environmental factors

4. Define the problem, determine the natural history, determine the extent of the problem, plan a control strategy, implement a control strategy, evaluate a control strategy, plan research.

5. C

6. B

7. A class of nursing students usually shares a common bond in the desire to graduate and practice nursing. The class members interact with one another and may take group action related to many issues, such as "nursing as a profession" or "the welfare of nurses."

■ CHAPTER 8

Review Questions

1. A family is two or more people who are emotionally involved with each other and live in close geographical proximity. Both the family and the individual must be assessed in order to achieve their ultimate health potential. (Pages 191-192)

2. Two approaches for understanding the family are the structural-functional and developmental approaches (Page 194)

3. The eight stages of Duvall's family life cycle are: married couple without children; childbearing family; families with preschool children; families with school-age children; families with teenagers; families launching young adults; middle-aged parents; and aging family members. (Page 198)

4. The developmental tasks of each stage of Duvall's family life cycle are:
    I. Establish mutually satisfying relationships and establish relationships with each other's families.
    II. Adjust to parenting.

III. Nurture children.

IV. Educate and socialize children.

V. Help children balance freedom and responsibility.

VI. Release children and develop spousal interests.

VII. Solidify marital relationship.

VIII. Adjust to multiple losses. (Page 198)

5. The Edmonds family is experiencing a situational crisis, a crisis of conflict involving a specific event. In this case, the event is the teenager's pregnancy. The goal of crisis intervention should be to help the family to (a) confront the crisis in manageable increments, (b) identify the facts to clarify the event, (c) find and accept help. In this case, help Jane to understand the pregnancy, help her identify someone in her family to confide in, and offer to talk to her mother with her. Advise her of the community resources that can assist with the pregnancy and the baby. (Page 198)

6. Reassure the Edmonds family about their ability to handle the crisis, provide concrete assistance, help the family to perceive the pregnancy realistically, offer appropriate support devices, and explore coping mechanisms. (Page 199)

7. The five characteristics of a healthy family are: mutual respect and support, open communication, shared problem solving, flexibility, and enhancement of personal growth. (Page 203)

8. Freedman and Heinrich identify these family health tasks as: (a) recognizing interruptions of health or development; (b) seeking health care; (c) managing health-related crises; (d) providing care to sick members of the family; (e) maintaining a home environment that promotes good health; and (f) maintaining relationships with health care providers for wellness and illness care. (Pages 202-203)

9. To assess a family, nurses collect data related to environment, family structure, and family function. (Page 203)

10. The nurse can facilitate Mrs. Scanlon's right to self-determination in health care by recognizing the family's right and responsibility to make health care choices and by providing the health information, resources, support and guidance that the family needs to make the appropriate choices. (Page 206)

Self-Examination Questions

1. True

2. False

3. False

4. True

5. Situational, maturational

6. Religious groups, kinship networks

■ CHAPTER 9

Review Questions

1. Culture is a pattern of learned behaviors and values that are shared among members of a designated group. To understand a client's view of life, the nurse must have knowledge of the client's culture (Page 212)

2. Culture is transmitted from generation to generation through enculturation. This is a process by which one learns appropriate ways of acting and meeting one's needs. (Page 212)

3. Answers will vary.

4. Ethnicity refers to affiliation with a group based on heredity and cultural traditions, such as language and religion. Race refers to a group of people who are descended from a common ancestor and possess common interests, appearance, or habits. (Page 213)

5. Nurses learn to become culturally sensitive by first becoming familiar with their own culture and understanding their culturally influenced values, beliefs, and behaviors. They also must become familiar with the values, beliefs, and practices of other cultures. Intercultural collaboration depends on the nurse's recognition that the client's cultural values, beliefs, and practices have relevance for care. Nurses who understand and respect a client's culture and are able to bridge cultural differences are able to provide culturally sensitive care. (Page 241)

6. Answers will vary. (Pages 220-221)

7. Spirituality is a belief in or relationship with a higher power, divine being, or creative life force. Religion refers to an organized system of worship with central beliefs, rituals, and practices. Many of the beliefs clients have regarding health and illness come from their religious or spiritual beliefs. The beliefs people have regarding health are closely linked to the actions they will take. (Page 233)

8. The nurse needs to assess how Mrs. Romonosky's religion affects her lifestyle, attitudes, and feelings about illness and health care. (Page 233)

9. The nurse should assess Mr. Salam's religious requirements. Black Muslims have dietary regulations restricting pork, shellfish, and certain vegetables. A diabetic Muslim will refuse porcine insulin because the pig is considered unclean. (Page 237)

10. The nurse should assess the religious needs of the Cohen family. In addition, in Orthodox Judaism, transplants and donation of body parts are prohibited. (Page 236)

Self-Examination Questions

1. Culture is: shared, learned, social, adaptive, relative.

2. Enculturation is the socialization of children into norms of their culture.

3. Acculturation is the cultural change that occurs in response to the prolonged contact of one culture with another.

4. Time orientation, territoriality, gender role behavior, aging, family

5. Ethnocentrism is the belief that one's culture or way of life is superior to that of another culture.

6. Culture shock is the psychological and social difficulty that individuals experience in adapting to a new culture.

■ **CHAPTER 10**

Review Questions

1. Individuality is the total character peculiar to an individual that distinguishes that individual from all other people.   The total character encompasses the whole of an individual's behavioral and emotional tendencies, including attitudes, habits, values, motives, abilities, appearance, and psychic state. It is important for nurses to understand clients as individuals because individuality influences the way a person thinks, feels, and acts in any given situation   (Page 248)

2. Maslow proposed a hierarchy of needs that consists of five different levels. As an individual passes through life there is movement up and down within this hierarchy as well as overlapping of needs, and specific needs change due to alterations in the human organism and the environment.   This concept assists nurses in understanding clients' needs and the reasons underlying clients' behaviors. It enables nurses to anticipate how a client might react to her or his health care. (Pages 249-250)

3. Self-actualized people have a firm foundation for development of a personal value system. They have a philosophical acceptance of themselves and their environment. They are able to discriminate between means and ends in terms of goal satisfaction. Conflict and struggle over choices lessen or disappear in many areas of life. Self-actualized people have the full use of their talents, capacities, and potential. (Page 251)

4. Body image, gender identity, self-esteem and role performance are components of self-concept. Each of the components develops and changes as an individual gains experience in her or his environment. (Page 254)

5. The nurse should anticipate concerns in the area of self-esteem, gender identity, self-concept and role performance. (Page 254)

6. According to Erikson, John is in the stage of transition between childhood and adulthood. Adolescents must accept a new body image and perform certain tasks relevant to establishing a sexual role, selecting an occupation, becoming independent of the family, and acquiring a social rather than egocentric response to others. Without successful mastery of these tasks, individuals may develop identity confusion. The nurse needs to assess these areas carefully with John. (Page 259)

7. During adolescence, both males and females become sexually mature. The gonads develop fully and secretions of androgens and estrogens are at peak levels. The capacity to respond quickly and repeatedly to sexual stimuli is common. The nurse will need to assess John's sexual development prior to hospitalization and work with him collaboratively in understanding the changes his injury will effect. (Page 270)

8. In order to gain sufficient information and understanding about a client's sexuality, a nurse needs to accept and understand his or her sexuality. Nurses need to learn to assess clients' personal attitudes about sexuality and life experiences without being judgmental or imposing their own values. Clarification of personal attitudes about sexual issues should enable nurses to address these needs in clients. (Page 271)

9. The nurse should respond to Miss Lambert that although changes occur due to aging, the changes are not equated with a cessation of sexual functioning or diminution of its importance. Sexual interest usually remains consistent throughout adulthood for both males and females. Some individuals report increased sexual interest and activity as they become older. (Page 270)

10. The nurse should discuss potential changes due to menopause, increased ability for physical and emotional intimacy, and conflicts about gender role and sex roles. (Page 269)

Self-Examination Questions

1. The total character peculiar to an individual, which distinguishes that individual from all others

2. B

3. C

4. Attitudes toward the self; growth, development, and self-actualization; integration; autonomy; perception of reality; and environment mastery

5. Early childhood transition, early adult transition, midlife transition, and late adult transition

6. B

■ CHAPTER 11

Review Questions

1. Openness and acceptance toward people of all ages; highly developed communication skills (verbal and nonverbal). (Pages 276-277)

2. Although frequently used synonymously, the terms growth and development refer to two very different processes. Growth describes physical changes in size, height, and weight from conception to about 18 years of age. Development describes changes in psychosocial, cognitive, or moral functioning. (Page 277)

3. A. Growth and development follow a predictable, continuous, and sequential pattern.
   B. Neuromuscular growth and development follow both cephalocaudal and proximodistal patterns.
   C. Each stage of development is dependent on completion of the previous stage and is itself the foundation for the development of new skills.
   D. Growth or development may be temporarily stalled or regress during critical periods.
   E. Individual variations depend on genetics, environment, and positive and negative factors present or absent during critical periods. (Page 279)

4. A. Neonate: Gains 5-7 ounces each week during first four weeks of life. (Page 282)
   B. Infant: Gains head control by 3 months. (Page 285)
   C. Toddler: Legs begin to lengthen. (Page 291)
   D. Preschooler: Develops fine motor skills. (Page 296)
   E. School-age child: Experiences eruption of permanent teeth. (Page 302)
   F. Adolescent: Both sexes experience a growth spurt. (Page 305)
   G. Young adult: Experiences rapid personal and social changes rather than physical growth. (Page 309)
   H. Middle-aged adult: Body weight redistributes around the waist, hips, and abdomen. (Page 313)
   I. Older adult: Experiences decreases in memory, hearing, vision, taste, and smell. (Page 315)

5. A. Neonate: Crying, looking, and reflex activities are primary means of expression. (Page 282)
   B. Infant: Further develops a pattern of trust versus mistrust. (Page 286)
   C. Toddler: Imitates the behaviors of significant people. (Page 292)
   D. Preschooler: Has a sense of curiosity and adventure and a desire to explore. (Page 296)

E. School-age child: Develops a pattern of industry versus inferiority. (Page 302)
F. Adolescent: The peer group becomes the primary influence. (Page 306)
G. Young adult: Choosing a career path and building personal relationships are foremost. (Page 309)
H. Middle-aged adult: Showing care for others in active and satisfying ways is a primary task. (Page 313)
I. Older adult: Develops perspective on life based on experience and has a desire to pass this on. (Page 316)

6. A. Neonate: colic, thrush (Page 283)
   B. Infant: infections, accidents (Page 288)
   C. Toddler: abuse and neglect, lead poisoning (Page 293)
   D. Preschooler: infections, obesity or malnutrition (Page 298)
   E. School-age child: dental health problems, learning disorders (Page 303)
   F. Adolescent: alcohol and drug abuse, sexually transmitted disease (Page 307)
   G. Young adult: stress, substance abuse (Page 311)
   H. Middle-aged adult: cancer, degenerative musculoskeletal disease (Page 315)
   I. Older adult: sleep disturbances, sensory deficits (Page 317)

7. The term maturation describes a differentiation or increasing complexity of capabilities that may come with age. (Page 277)

8. The Denver Developmental Screening Test (DDST) assesses the level of developmental maturity in infants and young children. The Vineland Social Maturity Scale assesses adaptive behavior and social readiness in school-age children. (Page 280)

9. Engage clients in a life review or reminiscence; explore alternative ways of adapting and coping with health problems; discuss the economics of health care, which are frequently overwhelming to adults on fixed incomes. (Page 319)

10. By 7-9 months; individuation (Page 287)

Self-Examination Questions

1. A and B

2. Therapeutic play is a way of assisting or encouraging children through play to express their feelings, fears, and conflicts so that they can master them.

3. B

4. True

5. False

6. Influence of genetic, environmental, and other factors during critical periods

7. Choice of career; choice of mate; independence from family of origin; establishment of sexual relationship and gender affiliation; religious, moral, and ethical standards; financial independence

8. Changes in visual acuity; decreased muscular agility and flexibility; changes in auditory acuity; changes in memory retention patterns; changes in energy level and stamina; changes in subcutaneous fat deposits affecting self-esteem and body image

- **CHAPTER 12**

Review Questions

1. The sick role is learned through being sick and interacting with family, community, and culture. It is a role that is not familiar to most people, is assumed with difficulty, and involves feelings and behaviors reflective of fear and anxiety about health states and mortality. (Page 330)

2. Right: exempt from daily responsibilities
   Obligation: expected to seek professional help in order to overcome the disease
   Right: absolved from any responsibility for the illness state
   Obligation: expected to articulate the desire to get well (Page 330)

3. The Szasz-Hollander model stresses that the client will take an active role in the provider-client relationship. (Page 331)

4. A. Stage: transition from self-perception of health to ill
      Client problem: denial
   B. Stage: accepts illness and seeks help
      Client problem: repression
   C. Stage: convalescence
      Client problem: hesitancy to leave the sick role. (Pages 332-333)

5. Threats to personal injury; altered body image; pain; separation from family, friends, and work; unrealistic expectations of staff; unfamiliarity with medical terminology (Page 334)

6. Fear; anxiety; hostility; acting out--physical and verbal abuse, uncontrollable crying, laughing, and screaming (Page 336)

7. Studies consistently demonstrate the increased health risk for persons with low quantity and quality of interpersonal relationships. (Page 327)

8. The holistic perspective of health acknowledges an individual's adaptation to the environment, emphasizes equal relationships between the nurse and the client, and supports collaboration, health maintenance, education, and the treatment of the entire person. (Page 324)

9. Sense of well-being; presence or absence of symptoms; ability to carry on with day-to-day responsibilities (Page 324)

10. Recognition of signs and symptoms; number and duration of symptoms; perceived seriousness of symptoms; functional interference; cultural and socioeconomic interpretation of symptoms (Pages 326-327)

Self-Examination Questions

1. Perceived susceptibility, perceived seriousness, perceived benefits of taking action and barriers to taking action, and cues to action.

2. B

3. True

4. In the collaborative relationship, the appropriate client role is an active one that exercises some degree of power in the provider-client relationship. The relationship is reciprocal in that the client is given and takes an active role in the care process.

5. C

■ CHAPTER 13

Review Questions

1. Friendly, understanding and emotionally stable; aware of personal values, feelings, motives, and goals; aware of personal strengths and limitations; sense of purpose in life; able to use a collaborative approach (Page 348)

2. The facilitation phase allows the client to describe problems without being judged. In the transition phase the nurse works with the client to define the problem and recognize mutual responsibility for the problem's solution. During the action phase, the nurse collaborates with the client to develop a plan to handle present problems and devise methods to deal with future problems. (Page 351-352)

3. A. Words are used to accurately state a client's feelings and convey understanding of the client's position about a particular situation.
    B. Belief in the client's ability to solve his or her own problems is demonstrated.
    C. Caring is demonstrated by use of gesture, tone of voice, touch, and facial expression.
    D. Responding directly to specific concerns expressed by clients and requesting clarification of vague or abstract statements.
    E. The helpers communicate in a constructive way that they mean what they say or do.
    F. Personal experiences with similar problems and solutions are shared with the client.
    G. The client is informed about discrepancies between what he or she has been saying or doing.
    H. Communicating with the client about the nurse-client relationship as it exists at that moment in time.
    I. Confidence that another will accept one for who one is and will respond genuinely.
    J. The capacity for self direction.
    K. The process of sharing with another person. (Pages 351-353)

4. Preinteraction phase--after reviewing or reading a record, the nurse begins to conceptualize some preliminary problems and goals for the client.
    Orientation phase--nurse and client establish mutual expectations, often based on a verbal contract.
    Working phase--the nurse and client engage in active problem solving.
    Termination phase--the formal nurse-client helping relationship is ended. (Pages 355-358)

5. A. True
    B. False. Sympathetic feelings for the other may preclude or prevent helpful action in a nonprofessional relationship. (Page 347)

6. A. Pets provide individuals with outlets for nurturant needs and can help to relieve loneliness and isolation.
    B. Individuals such as Mother Teresa dedicate their life to the furthering of one's particular belief or cause.
    C. A continuum, from absence of concern about spiritual entities to a strong sense of and need for faith.
    D. An interpersonal relationship is a social relationship that occurs among people within a marriage, family, friendship, school, business, church, or health care setting. (Page 346)

7. Trust (Page 352)

8. Comfortable with increasing self-awareness and able to share this awareness with others; open to differences in others; welcomes new experiences; future oriented; able to postpone gratification of immediate needs for larger goals (Page 352)

9. The helping relationship (Page 350)

10. Collaboration moves the relationship in the direction of meeting client needs and goals. It encourages the client to take a much more active role. It places the nurse and the client in a partnership role. (Page 350)

Self-Examination Questions

1. (1) c, (2) d, (3) a, (4) b, (5) g, (6) h, (7) f, (8) e

2. False

3. False

4. True

5. B

6. B

7. D

8. (1) N, (2) P, (3) P, (4) N

■ **CHAPTER 14**

Review Questions

1. Communication: all the processes by which people influence each other (Page 364)

2. A. Context, or setting and circumstances, in which the communication takes place
    B. Sender of the message, which includes the anatomical structures and physiological processes necessary for thinking and speech
    C. Message, which includes the verbal and nonverbal behaviors such as choice of words, tone of voice, and body language
    D. Receiver of the message, including all the senses used to do this
    E. Feedback, which is both the external message sent and the internal messages heard by both the receiver and the sender (such as fatigue, hunger, restlessness, anxiety, and boredom) (Pages 365-366)

3. A. Perception--the ability to correctly interpret the actual message being sent
    B. Evaluation--the ability to analyze the message that has been sent
    C. Transmission--the actual expression of the message from the sender to the receiver (Page 366)

4. Teaching; facilitating expression of feelings; alleviating anxiety and fear; promoting problem-solving; asserting a point of view (Pages 372-373)

5. Listening can be a very empowering response in communication. It is an active process in which the listener focuses on the speaker's message and responds with attention, warmth, empathy, and respect for what is being said. (Page 373).

6. Approaches that support communication: empathy, genuineness, self-disclosure, immediacy. (Pages 374-379) Approaches that hinder communication: failure to listen, lack of probing, being judgmental, false reassurances. (Page 381)

7. An informal interview is direct and seeks to obtain the most important information in a timely manner. It usually is conducted in a clinic, home, or school nurse's office. A formal interview is longer and more structured than the informal interview. Often a printed form, checklist, or outline is used in order to obtain complete and comprehensive data. (Pages 385-386)

8. A. Establish verbal contact with the client giving name, title, role, purpose of the interview, time involved, and protection of confidentiality.
   B. Choose a private setting free from distractions.
   C. Vary your approach to accommodate client's needs.
   D. Balance the use of direct and indirect open-ended questions.
   E. Collect only data that are not available elsewhere.
   F. Respect the client's right to refuse to provide information.
   G. Summarize the information collected.
   H. Bring closure to the interview. (Page 386)

9. A. Repeat your message in different ways rather than speaking louder.
   B. Prepare preschool children by allowing them to touch objects involved, carrying out the procedure on a doll, or using play to reenact the event after it is done.
   C. Use the client's language to communicate with simple words or use an interpreter. (Page 383)

10. A. Verbal communication includes language and the meaning of words as well as physiological and cognitive mechanisms necessary for speech and hearing.
    B. Nonverbal communication includes all forms of communication that do not involve words, such as posture and gait, facial expression, eye contact, hand gestures, tone of voice, and use or nonuse of touch.
    C. Metacommunication describes the total impact of the verbal and nonverbal messages individuals use. (Page 367)

Self-Examination Questions

1. (1) d, (2) c, (3) e, (4) a, (5) b

2. (1) a, (2) b, (3) d, (4) c, (5) b, (6) d, (7) a

3. (1) F, (2) T, (3) T, (4) T, (5) F

4. (1) c, (2) d, (3) a, (4) b, (5) e

■ CHAPTER 15

Review Questions

1. Professional decision-making is a methodical, systematic way of acquiring and combining information to make choices from a set of alternatives. (Page 391)

2. The activities of a systematic, deliberative process such as the nursing process include: identification, selection, and evaluation of essential information for making a decision; comparison of the current situation with prior knowledge and experiences to gain insight about the decisions that must be made; seeking out appropriate resources to assist in the decision process. (Page 392)

3. Nonsystematic approaches to decision-making include:
   Tradition--based on beliefs, values, customs, or norms that have been handed down over time (taking vital signs at the beginning of the shift each day).
   Trial and error--one or more interventions are tried until something succeeds in improving the situation (treating pressure sores with two or three approaches until one works rather than basing the approach on current literature and research).
   Habit--nurses use prior decision behaviors to make choices for current client situations without deliberating on their appropriateness for new situations (selecting an intervention to relieve pain before assessing the client). (Pages 392-393)

4. The two phases of the Berger-Williams model are assessment and management. (Page 394)

5. The six steps of the Berger-Williams model are data collection, data analysis, nursing diagnosis, planning, implementation, and evaluation. (Page 395)

6. Inductive reasoning is thinking that moves from particular facts to a general principle. For example, a nurse collects information and then makes a hypothesis. In deductive reasoning, thinking moves from general principles to the collection of specific data. For example, a nurse makes a nursing diagnosis and then collects information to confirm or negate it. (Page 395)

7. Inductive reasoning is not superior to deductive reasoning. Although useful in some situations, inductive reasoning has a serious limitation: information overload, which can lead to subsequent errors in judgment. (Page 395)

8. A. Determine the importance (essential, contributory, noncontributory) of the data.
   B. Evaluate the type of measurement used in collecting the data.
   C. Evaluate the source of the data for appropriateness and accuracy. (Page 396)

9. A. Bayes' theorem: a statistical method used for making clinical diagnostic judgments based on the rate of incidence of the diagnosis, the probability of clinical cues occurring, and the probability of a cue given a certain diagnosis.
   B. Decision trees: a branching diagram of various alternative choices and outcomes.
   C. Decision matrix: a pictorial organization of possible alternative choices and outcomes.
   D. Networks: the critical path method in which a care plan with a timeline is developed. (Pages 401-405)

10. Expertise in decision making; biases; values, attitudes, and beliefs; risk-taking behaviors; comfort level; communication skills (Pages 405-408)

Self-Examination Questions

1. c

2. d

3. a

4. c

5. b

6. True

■ **CHAPTER 16**

Review Questions

1. Greet Mr. R. in the hallway and introduce yourself by name as the nurse who will be taking care of him. Accompany him to the examination room, making sure he knows where he is and what is going on. Tell him how to get help should he need it. Tell him you will be back as soon as you can to help him undress and to get on the exam table. Reassure him that his daughter will be coming soon. (Pages 419-420)

2. A. Put Mr. R. in a room to wait rather than letting him wait in the hallway (privacy).
   B. Introduce yourself by name as the nurse who will be caring for him (emotional comfort).
   C. Make sure he understands what is going on (decreased anxiety).
   D. Assure him that he can get help when he needs it (client control).
   E. Make sure that he is comfortable before leaving him alone in the room (comfort). (Pages 419-420)

3. A. "I don't remember what happened!"
   B. "I was getting up from the kitchen chair, and the next thing I knew I as on the floor."
   C. "My left hand feels sort of tingly." (Page 418)

4. A. While helping Mr. R to undress, inspect his overall state of health.
   B. Look for signs of distress as you help Mr. R. onto the exam table.
   C. Observe Mr. R.'s vital signs, facial expressions, body size, and appearance as part of a nutritional assessment. (Page 418)

5. A. "Describe what you eat in a normal day."
   B. "Tell me more about that." (Page 423)

6. "Is there anything you would like to discuss that I have not yet asked you about?" (Page 423)

7. Inspection and palpation provide an overall impression of the client's present state of health. (Page 436)

8. Direct percussion consists of tapping an area directly with the fingertip of the middle finger or thumb. Indirect percussion interposes a finger between the area to be percussed and the finger creating the vibrations. (Page 437)

9. A. The stethoscope bell is used to auscultate low-frequency sounds.
    B. The stethoscope diaphragm is used to auscultate high-frequency sounds. (Page 438)

10. A. "What has your doctor told you about your health."
    B. "Can you tell me your full name? What is today's date? Where are you right now?"
    C. "Describe the last time you learned something new." (Page 427)

11. Height; weight; head circumference; limb length; limb circumference; body temperature; respiration; pulse; blood pressure (Pages 439-487)

12. Heat production and conservation: basal metabolic rate; muscle activity; hormone secretion; circadian rhythm. Heat loss: conduction; convection; radiation; evaporation; diurnal fluctuations; exercise habits; stress; age; environmental temperature and humidity (Page 443-446)

13. Age and gender; disease; metabolism; stress; medications; environment, including altitude, air pollution, and environmental temperature (Pages 461-462)

14. Pulse rate; pulse rhythm; pulse volume/amplitude; pulse symmetry (Page 465)

15. Systolic blood pressure is the pressure exerted against the arterial wall as the left ventricle contracts and forces blood into the aorta. It is the maximum pressure that is exerted against the vessel wall. Diastolic pressure is the arterial pressure that is measured as the left ventricle relaxes and the heart is at rest. It is the minimal constant arterial wall pressure. (Page 473)

16. General assessment refers to a broad overview of the physical appearance and demeanor of the client. Among the observations the nurse makes are overall impressions of mental status, speech, body development (height and weight) and posture, movement, gait, and energy level. (Page 487)

17. Inspection; palpation; percussion; auscultation (Page 436-438)

18. See text pages 492-567, including Tables 16-13 and 16-16 through 16-45.

Self-Examination Questions

1. The lower edge of blood pressure cuff should be placed 2.5 cm (1 inch) above the antecubital fossa, with the cuff bladder centered over the brachial artery.

2. The formula for converting Fahrenheit to centigrade is F - 32 x 5/9 = C. The answer is 37.8° C.

3. D

4. Two nurses are required to perform the procedure.

5. Primary concern; current understanding; history of past health problems/experiences; personal, family, and social history; subjective manifestations

■ **CHAPTER 17**

Review Questions

1. A nursing problem or diagnosis describes a health condition primarily resolved by nursing interventions or therapies--for example, pain and discomfort or impaired functioning in such areas as rest, sleep, ventilation, circulation, activity, nutrition, and patterns of elimination. Asthma and breast cancer are two examples of medical problems or diagnoses. Neither is directly preventable by nursing therapies and both are referred to physicians once they become a medical condition (Page 581)

2. Nursing diagnosis is the diagnostic reasoning part of the nursing process. (Page 576)

3. Development of the North American Nursing Diagnosis Association (NANDA) (Page 574)

4. A classification system that organizes classes of phenomena into a hierarchical structure and helps direct the discovery of new information. A familiar example can be found in zoology, where animals are classified according to kingdom, phylum, class, order, family, genus, and species. (Page 576)

5. A. Statement of the client's actual or potential health problem or health state (for example, impaired skin integrity)
   B. The etiology, or related/contributing factors (for example, impaired skin integrity due to nutritional deficit)
   C. Signs and symptoms (for example, impaired skin integrity with destruction of skin layers) (Pages 577-578)

6. A. Pain R/T surgical incision AEB: client statements such as "it hurts"
   B. Constipation R/T immobility AEB: no BM x 5 days
   C. Activity intolerance R/T hypoxemia AEB: pallor, heart rate of 30 BPM
   D. Self-esteem disturbance R/T recent divorce AEB: client statements such as "who cares?"

7. Actual nursing diagnoses such as pain, sleep disturbances, or self-care limitations have already been defined by the nurse based on the client's responses. Potential nursing diagnoses require the nurse to identify client risk factors for a particular problem. (Page 580).

8. A cue is a raw piece of information, such as sweaty palms or restlessness. An inference is the assignment of meaning to clustered cues, such as anxiety. (Page 585)

9. The most common type of diagnostic error is the inferential leap. It consists of making premature conclusions based on too early termination of either the data gathering or the data analysis phase of the nursing process. Frequent studies have shown that the novice will conduct insufficient data gathering whereas the expert will perform insufficient data analysis. (Page 587)

10. A. Aids in identifying and describing the domain and scope of nursing practice.
    B. Focuses nursing care on the client's response to problems.
    C. Facilitates the evaluation of nursing practice.
    D. Provides a framework for testing the validity of nursing interventions.
    E. Prescribes the content of nursing curriculum.
    F. Leads to more comprehensive and individualized client care. (Page 588)

Enrichment Activities

Case Study 1

1. Knowledge Deficit: Management and implications of DM R/T lack of exposure and information misinterpretation.

2. Fear: Unacceptable dietary restrictions, self-injection, and possibly death R/T recent medical diagnosis of DM; misinterpretation of life-style implications AEB: "I'm so scared," tearfulness.

3. Altered Nutrition: More Than Body Carbohydrate (CHO) Requirements R/T pathophysiologic alteration in CHO metabolism, insufficient physical exercise, eating in response to internal cues other than hunger (i.e., anxiety, need gratification) AEB: FBS 400, wt 20% over ideal for height and frame.

4. Ineffective Individual Coping R/T situational crisis (recent diagnosis of DM), personal vulnerability (lack of interpersonal support system) AEB: tearfulness, perceived powerlessness, compromised problem solving.

Case Study 2

1. Pain R/T surgical incision AEB: pinched brow, facial mask of pain, reluctance to move or reposition.

2. Ineffective Breathing Pattern R/T pain from high abdominal incision, refusal to participate in deep breathing, obesity AEB: respirations 24 at rest, shallow and asymmetrical breathing, crackles R lung base.

3. Potential for Constipation R/T general anesthesia, relative immobility, nonparticipation in physical exercise regime, NPO.

4. Potential for Ineffective Airway Clearance R/T excessive mucus secretion and impaired mucus mobility secondary to 60-pack-year smoking history, pain, ineffective breathing pattern.

Self-Examination Questions

1. Refer to Box 17-2, page 576.

2. A

3. True

4. False

5. Problem, etiology, signs and symptoms (defining characteristics)

6. A. No. A medical diagnosis.
    B. No. Not on approved list. Also, anorexia is a symptom, in this case of the diagnosis Altered Nutrition: Potential for Less Than Body RDA Requirements, Risk Factor: chemotherapy side effects.
    C. No. This is a technical problem, needing technical intervention, but not a nursing diagnosis.
    D. Yes.
    E. Yes. Salt substitutes are quite high in potassium.
    F. OK, but relationship not directly clear. What about Activity Intolerance R/T decreased cardiac output; or Impaired Home Maintenance Management R/T activity intolerance?
    G. Yes.
    H. Fear of what? Needs to be made specific before treatment can be planned.

■ **CHAPTER 18**

Review Questions

1. A. Describes the expected client status when a nursing diagnosis has been resolved.
   B. The collective activities that a nurse and a client select to correct or alleviate the health problem identified in the nursing diagnosis statement.
   C. Statements that describe acceptable evidence that outcomes have been achieved. (Page 592)

2. A. Incorporate clients' and nurses' concepts and values of health.
   B. Address clients' primary concerns.
   C. Draw from clients' own resources and capabilities.
   D. Communicate nurses' respect and empower clients.
   E. Reflect clients' values and informed consent.
   F. Enhance clients' motivation to carry out the plan. (Page 592)

3. A. Determine the urgency of the client's needs through use of a framework such as Maslow's hierarchy of needs.
   B. Elicit and understand the client's beliefs, values, desires, and perceptions of his or her needs.
   C. Explore available resources and services.
   D. Identify situational variables, such as diagnostic tests or special procedures that may take special precedence. (Pages 595-596)

4. Nature of the client's problem; client's resources, such as personal strengths, support persons, environment, and finances; and realistic expectations (Page 597)

5. Describe client behavior, status, functioning, or condition; use positive terms; relate each desired outcome statement to only one nursing diagnosis; specify the expected time frame for outcome attainment. (Page 601)

6. Long-term outcomes describe complete resolution of a problem in broad, global terms (for example, healthy bowel elimination pattern). Short-term outcomes relate to more immediate changes in client status and frequently represent steps toward long-term outcomes (for example, client's knowledge of behaviors that promote a healthy bowel elimination pattern). (Pages 596-597)

7. A. Monitoring is the ongoing collection of data about a client's condition and includes listening.
   B. Analyzing examines client achievement of or progress toward desired outcomes.
   C. Collaborating involves nurse-client discussion of the results of the nurse's analysis and leads to the client and nurse reaching a mutual conclusion about whether further action is needed.
   D. Deciding is the mutual determination by nurse and client about terminating, continuing, or modifying the plan of care. (Pages 610-612)

8. A. Focused: Identify the client by name, room number, primary physician, and admitting diagnosis.
   B. Orderly: All information relevant to one client is provided before moving on to additional clients or topics.
   C. Precise: Use terminology that clearly describes the event or situation.
   D. Concise: Include pertinent information only, not extraneous details.
   E. Comprehensive: Provide all relevant data necessary to give an accurate account of a situation or event. (Page 613)

9. A. Formative evaluation determines client progress toward desired outcomes and helps the nurse identify and correct patterns contributing to a lack of progress.

B. Summative evaluation determines whether outcomes were met, partially met, or not met. Failure to achieve outcomes by target dates indicate the quality of the plan and the formative evaluation process were inadequate. (Page 610)

10. The purpose is to assess the quality of health services provided throughout an entire health care agency. The steps include: selecting the topic, identifying standards and criteria, collecting data, interpreting data, selecting and implementing solutions, and reevaluating. (Pages 625-626)

Self-Examination Questions

1. Formulating desired outcomes and outcome criteria, identifying priorities, defining nursing implementation to meet goals, and developing evaluation criteria

2. E

3. The difference is the point in time at which they are conducted. Formative--ongoing activity; provides continuous feedback about progress toward desired outcomes. Summative--occurs at target date or on discharge; determines to what extent desired outcomes have been met. Retrospective--occurs after discharge or after termination of care; determines whether desired outcomes have been met and whether discharge needs were planned and provisions made

4. Relate each outcome statement to one nursing diagnosis only; designate the subject; use action verbs to describe specific, measurable client behaviors; state outcomes in positive terms; and include conditions under which behavior is expected to occur.

5. D

6. Subject, action verb, content focus, and time

■ CHAPTER 19

Review Questions

1. Two or more members, interplay between members, common objectives, common rules, specific roles and responsibilities for members, and a sense of cohesion among members (Page 632)

2. A. Dependence: Members get to know each other.
    B. Independence: Characterized by development of a group identity, group structure, and roles of members.
    C. Interdependence: The group moves toward its goals and stimulates productivity. (Page 633-634)

3. The primary role of the health care team is meeting the health care needs of clients through information sharing, efficient and comprehensive care planning, prevention of complications, and continuity of care.

Collaborative functions: registered nurse--diagnose and treat human response to actual or potential health problems; physical/occupational therapist--assist clients to attain optimum musculoskeletal functioning after injury, illness, or surgery; social worker--focus on discharge planning, referrals to community agencies, and client and family counseling; dietician--assist clients and families in nutritional counseling and therapy; chaplain--assist clients and families in meeting their spiritual needs; pharmacist--dispense medication prescribed by physicians, psychiatrists, dentists, and nurse practitioners; physician--diagnose and treat medical conditions or problems (Pages 637-642)

4. Working together toward common goals in a cooperative manner; recognizing the unique contribution of each member in a working relationship (Page 637)

5. The role of the initiator is primarily task oriented. The initiator introduces objectives, requests information, presents ideas or facts, clarifies information, summarizes, focuses the group on the task at hand, and reacts constructively to the ideas of others.

   The role of the maintainer is to foster good group dynamics. The maintainer recognizes contributions; appeases differences; shares perceptions, attitudes, opinions, and emotions; and compromises his or her own stance to facilitate group cohesiveness. (Page 647)

6. The nurse can perform the role of the initiator by proposing new ideas, clarifying team decisions, and evaluating the effectiveness of the care plan. As maintainer, the nurse can lead team conferences, plan discharges or act as a consultant. (Page 648)

7. A. Assertiveness: Express confidence that one's ideas and rights are important.
   B. Risk taking: Take action or state a value that is outside of the prevailing group norm.
   C. Accountability: Assume responsibility for one's actions and decisions.
   D. Autonomy: Accept freedom to choose one's actions. (Page 649)

8. Traditional top-down communication, territoriality, interprofessional communication problems, ambiguity of expectations, and differences in education (Pages 650-651)

9. Extrinsic: Mutual respect, clarity of roles, open lines of communication, joint educational experiences
   Intrinsic: Maturity/self-confidence, accountability for own actions, clinical competence, willingness to accept change. (Page 649)

10. Conflicting professional values of individual team members; changing nature of today's health care system (Page 652)

Self-Examination Questions

1. A

2. C

3. Disease/illness phenomena; responses to actual or potential health problems

4. D

5. C

6. A

■ **CHAPTER 20**

Review Questions

1. Learning is a continuous process in which a person's behavior is modified by experience. It takes place with or without teaching effort. Teaching attempts to influence learning toward specific goals. (Pages 657-658)

2. A. The Patient Bill of Rights
    B. The doctrine of informed consent
    C. The consumer movement
    D. Increase in chronic illness
    E. Emphasis on health promotion
    F. Health care payment systems (Pages 658-659)

3. A. Professional standards
    B. Nurse Practice Acts
    C. Professional literature (Page 659)

4. (1) c, (2) d, (3) a, (4) b   (Pages 662-664)

5. Functionally illiterate individuals cannot cope with the minimal reading requirements of everyday life. (Page 670)

6. A. Lack of exposure
    B. Lack of recall
    C. Information misinterpretation
    D. Cognitive limitations
    E. Lack of interest in learning
    F. Unfamiliarity with information resources (Page 675)

7. A. Motivation
    B. Health beliefs
    C. Past learning experiences
    D. Emotional status
    E. Physical condition
    F. Developmental stage (Pages 666-668)

8. A. Readiness
    B. Ability
    C. Learning styles (Page 666)

9. (1) f, (2) e, (3) d, (4) c, (5) b, (6) a (Pages 684-686)

10. A. Facilitative teaching behaviors
    B. Giving feedback
    C. Providing positive reinforcement
    D. Using prompts
    E. Practice and repetition
    F. Facilitating transfer of learning (Pages 687-688)

Self-Examination Questions

1. (1) c, (2) d, (3) b, (4) a, (5) b

2. D

■ CHAPTER 21

Review Questions

1. Admissions, discharge and transfer; nursing assessments; client care plans; client teaching plans; clinical reference retrievals (Pages 704-707)

2. Greater timeliness of client information data; increased accuracy of documentation; improved legibility of assessments, care plans and shift reports; easier access to client data for decision making by other health care personnel (Pages 709-710)

3. Lack of client security; lack of client confidentiality; unauthorized access (Page 710)

4. (1) d, (2) c, (3) b, (4) a

5. Computerized literature searches; note collection and data analysis; research aids in sorting results (Page 716)

6. Patient classification systems; staff scheduling systems; inventory systems; personnel files (Page 717)

7. Word processing for changing and updating policy and procedure manuals; electronic spreadsheets for performing mathematical calculations; data base management systems for creating computerized filing systems (Page 718)

8. The HELP (Health Evaluation Through Logical Processing) System assists in decision making by giving nurses treatment protocols and warnings. For the family, if a client has an elevated potassium level and is receiving potassium supplements orally, a warning alert is printed. (Page 711)

9. NLN annual *Directory of Educational Software,* which reviews and rates the available programs; the annual software exchange list published in the March/April issue of *Computers in Nursing,* which does not review or rate the programs (Page 715)

10. MEDLARS (Medical Literature Analysis and Retrieval System)--twenty available online databases from the National Library of Medicine
    MEDLINE (Medical Literature Analysis and Retrieval System On-Line)--one of the world's largest bibliographic data bases of medical information; simultaneously searches listings in the *Index Medicus, International Nursing Index* and the *Index to Dental Literature*
    CINAHL (Cumulative Index to Nursing and Allied Health Literature)--includes some journals and magazines not referenced in the *International Nursing Index* (Page 716)

Self-Examination Questions

1. C

2. C

3. C

4. D

5. B

6.   C

7.   B

■ **CHAPTER 22**

Review Questions

1.   1950s: Halbert L. Dunn--the concept of "high-level wellness; 1974: Canadian Ministry of Health and Welfare --*A New Perspective on the Health of Canadians;* 1977: Senate Select Committee on Nutrition and Human Needs--*Dietary Goals for the United States*; 1979: Department of Health, Education, and Welfare--*Healthy People* (Pages 726-727)

2.   The focus of nursing on wellness began with Florence Nightingale.   In 1974 Cynthia Oelbaum identified behaviors of optimal wellness in adults.   Barbara Blattner developed the holistic nursing model.   Nola Pender's model focuses on factors that influence an individual to attain well-being.   Carolyn C. Clark described the concept of "wellness nursing." (Pages 728-729)

3.   Elements of wellness life-style: eating well, being fit, feeling good, caring for herself and others, fitting in, being responsible   (Page 730-733)

4.   Hospitalization leads to loss of autonomy, loss of privacy, sensory alterations, social isolation, risks, pain and discomfort, and changes in body image and self-esteem (Pages 744-747)

5.   Universal precautions would be required in the ER.   If the client is admitted and the HIV status is negative, Tuberculosis Isolation would be the precaution of choice.   (Pages 787-788)

6.   You should ask someone else to bring the sponges to you.   Once a sterile field is opened it should never be unattended.   An alternative would be to cover it with a sterile drape while you retrieve the sponges and reglove.   (Page 801)

7.   The "five rights"--right drug, right dose, right time, right route, right client   (Pages 819-820)

8.   Record the time, date, and location of injection; name and amount of medication.   You must also check on immediate response and record if pertinent.   (Page 851)

9.   Assess the IV site for redness, swelling, warmth, and tenderness (indicators of inflammation)   (Page 858)

10. The immediate postoperative client must be assessed for respiratory status, cardiovascular status, neurological status, fluid balance, wound condition, comfort, and safety.   (Page 868)

Self-Examination Questions

1.   To eat well, one needs to select and ingest foods that provide appropriate nourishment and satisfaction.   One should eat a variety of foods, maintain a healthy weight, choose a diet low in fat and cholesterol, eat plenty of vegetables and grain products, use sugars in moderation, use salt in moderation, drink alcohol in moderation.

2.   Regular exercise contributes to a positive sense of well-being, including the specific benefits of increased energy, reduced fatigue, fewer bodily aches and pains, fewer colds, increased resistance to disease, improved self-esteem, improved sleep, increased self-confidence, enhanced sexual vitality.

3. D

4. Anxiety, fear, depression, powerlessness, loneliness, emotional conflict, dissatisfaction, pain, fatigue

5. Smoking, alcohol and drug abuse, unsafe sexual activity

6. Culture shock, loss of autonomy, loss of privacy, sensory overload or deprivation, social isolation, exposure to nosocomial infection, exposure to risks, exposure to pain and discomfort

7. Disruption in skin integrity and circulation, altered respiration, altered nutrition, altered elimination, decreased mobility, altered body temperature, sleep pattern disturbance, altered comfort, fluid and electrolyte imbalance, altered sensory perception, altered body image, altered role performance, self-care deficit, fear and anxiety

■ CHAPTER 23

Review Questions

1. Allison: pregnant woman, wife, mother, daughter, nurse; Bill: husband, father, son-in-law, policeman, student; Jenny: daughter, granddaughter, expectant sister; Betty: mother, grandmother, mother-in-law, caretaker (Page 890)

2. Caring involves self-expression and is based on equity. This is a process of give and take that incorporates the mutual sharing of self.   This means client participation in decisions about care, shared control of the professional relationship through mutual negotiation, self-disclosure, mutual learning, shared language, humor, and personal space. (Page 892)

3. Age, personality, neurosensory variables, sociocultural and economic variables, personal values and philosophy, health and illness, stress, medication and substance use, sex and sexuality (Pages 898-905)

4. Shock and disbelief; yearning and protest; anguish, disorganization, and despair; identification; reorganization. Allison is in the reorganization phase, living with the memories. (Pages 913-914)

5. Self-Esteem Disturbance is a negative self-evaluation about self or capabilities. It can have many sources, and the client may have no sense of belonging, no sense of competence, or no sense of worth. Look for self-negating comments, expressions of shame or guilt, rationalizations, inability to accept positive statements from others, projection of blame or responsibility onto others. Self-presentation may include poor eye contact, lack of attention to grooming and dress, and substance abuse. (Page 927)

6. Self-expression regarding sexuality, sexuality in later life, etiology of sexual dysfunction (Pages 932-933)

7. Self-esteem and self-expression are necessary considerations throughout the life span.   Identification of risk factors and stressors are necessary to prevent problems. Birth of a new baby and sibling may cause a crisis. (Pages 936-939)

8. Provide time and opportunity for self-disclosure about the threats to self-expression. Anxiety may also be reduced by explaining hospital routines, procedures, and tests and encouraging as much choice as possible by the client. (Page 948)

9. Chronic illnesses are generally incurable and long-lasting. These clients face loss of health; body image changes; self-esteem changes; loss of changes in relationships and roles; changes in life-style activities, leisure pursuits, and sexual functioning; loss of income, independence, and mastery over their environment. (Page 953)

10. Anger is a common and normal response during stressful periods. Clients may not be aware of how angry they are and nurses can help them understand this. Guidelines include: give client permission to express anger, point out that it is a normal response, help identify signs of anger, explore reasons for anger, help client distinguish appropriate expressions of anger, give time to verbalize and describe anger, do not use a counter response of anger toward the client. (Page 955)

Self-Examination Questions

1. Self-expression is the process by which a person's self-understanding is shared with others.

2. The public self is the self that is represented to others through one's situation and manner of behavior. The private self is the way one understands oneself to be, although others may not always agree.

3. The deepest values and commitments

4. Making a choice is an act of manifesting a personal preference. Preferences are an integral aspect of inner emotions and express a relationship between the object and the individual's inner world. For choices to be considered expressive, the individual must be able to choose freely and must be free from coercion, manipulation, or undue influence.

5. B and D

6. Caring involves mutual self-expression to achieve therapeutic reciprocity.

7. Disclosure is to distress what fever is to infection. Both are a sign of disturbance and a part of the restorative process.

8. Catharsis is the process of psychologically purging emotion, of "getting it off my chest."

9. Excitement, plateau, orgasm, resolution

10. Denial of illness is an adaptive maneuver by which individuals unknowingly try to reduce anxiety associated with illness by acting as though the illness did not exist.

■ CHAPTER 24

Review Questions

1. Burns are injuries due to heat, radiation, chemicals, or electricity. Thermal and electrical burns are classified by degrees, depending on the depth of the tissue injury. First-degree burns injure only the outer epidermis; second-degree burns extend into the dermis, causing blisters; third-degree burns destroy epidermis and dermis and damage underlying tissue. (Page 977)

2. Redness, heat, swelling, pain, and loss of function (Page 980)

3. The healing process consists of three overlapping phases: inflammation, proliferation, and maturation. Inflammation is a nonspecific defensive response to injury. Proliferation restores function of the injured area

and initiates tissue reconstruction.   Maturation involves reorganization and remodeling of the scar and can last several months. (Pages 980-981)

4.   Immature organ function creates some differences, especially in early infancy. Children have greater capacity for tissue repair, but they lack reserves and thereby are more vulnerable to electrolyte imbalance, body temperature fluctuation, and rapid spread of infection.   Infants' immature circulatory, respiratory, and neurological systems may impair healing. Infants have minimal energy stores and therefore malnutrition would compromise healing.   (Page 985)

5.   There can be many causes of skin lesions. It is helpful to explore the client's thoughts about the cause, what the client has done to treat the lesion, and the results. Explore environmental factors, time of appearance, past episodes, other problems associated with the lesion, and any changes before or after treatment. (Page 987)

6.   Impaired tissue integrity related to: altered circulation, nutritional deficit, fluid deficit or excess, knowledge deficit, impaired physical mobility, chemical irritants, thermal extremes, mechanical forces, radiation. Impaired skin integrity related to: mechanical factors, restraint, developmental factors. (Pages 993-996)

7.   The purpose of a bed bath is to clean the skin, promote circulation, relax muscles, and promote comfort and well-being. It also provides a good opportunity for complete integumentary assessment. The procedure should be discussed and mutually agreed upon with the client. Assemble equipment, prepare bed, prepare client (maintaining privacy), correct temperature of water, use soap sparingly, rinse and dry thoroughly. Start with head and face and proceed downward doing extremities, back, and genitalia. Provide clean linen and record. (Pages 1016-1021)

8.   Hands should be washed at the start. A clean glove is used to remove old dressing to protect the nurse. When the dressing is discarded and the equipment is prepared, a sterile glove is used on the hand that will be contacting the wound and the new dressing to protect the client from contamination and infection. (Pages 1042-1045)

9.   To detect and identify wound pathogens so that definitive therapy can be instituted. Culture is usually obtained during wound care when suspicious drainage or appearance is noted. (Page 1054)

10. Clarke and Kadhom reviewed research on pressure ulcers. They found that duration of pressure is a factor in ulcer generation and that relief of pressure is important to prevention. The time and frequency of nursing care of pressure ulcers significantly relates to prevention and is a nursing function. (Page 1060)

Self-Examination Questions

1.   C

2.   Noncellular connective tissue, elastin fibers, ground substances

3.   Protection, temperature regulation, sensation, excretion, lubrications

4.   F

5.   Vitamin C, vitamin A, vitamin B_6, niacin, riboflavin, thiamine

6.   B

7.   An ecchymosis, a term synonymous with bruise, represents diffuse bleeding into the tissue without encapsulation. A hematoma results when bleeding becomes encapsulated.

8. Epithelialization refers to the reproduction and migration of cells from the edge of the wound toward its center. New epithelial cells continue to form until the surface of the injury is covered.

9. This is the type of healing that occurs in wounds in which there is an actual loss of tissue. Replacement of the lost tissue requires prolonged healing time, and there is a more vigorous process of phagocytosis, which is necessary to remove debris and necrotic tissue.

10. A

■ **CHAPTER 25**

Review Questions

1. Energy balance refers to the amount of energy input relative to the amount of energy output in a given system (energy balance = energy input - energy output). A positive energy balance occurs when input exceeds output. Factors that influence energy input include type of food and the body's stores of energy. Energy output is influenced by basal metabolism rate and amount of physical activity. To maintain daily energy balance, the energy intake in the form of food must equal expenditure for basal metabolism, physical activity, and the energy used for food digestion, absorption, and transport. (Page 1069)

2. The six major classes of nutrients are carbohydrates, proteins, fats, vitamins, minerals, and water. (Page 1070)

3. Digestion--breakdown of foods into smaller compounds that can be absorbed into body fluids. Digestion involves both mechanical and chemical activity.
    Absorption--the process by which the end products of digestion are transferred from the lumen of the intestine to the circulatory system. The large molecules of protein, fats, and carbohydrates must be completely broken down into their smallest components before absorption can occur.
    Metabolism--the cellular process by which absorbed nutrients are used for cellular maintenance and energy production. The ultimate biological purpose of food ingestion is to support those metabolic processes that are essential to the life of the organism. (Page 1073-1078)

4. Factors that affect the nutritional status are the environment, age and health status. (Page 1080)

5. Kwashiorkor--malnutrition that develops when babies are weaned from the mother's milk without receiving a diet adequate in protein. The resulting protein deficiency creates a syndrome of retarded mental and physical growth, apathy, edema, muscular wasting, and skin depigmentation and dermatosis. Nurses should look for these signs in infants. (Page 1089)
    Marasmus--syndrome resulting from a deficiency of both protein and calories. The result is a general starvation and gross underweight. Edema is minimal and diarrhea is frequent. (Page 1089)
    Protein deficiency state--a protein deficiency malnutrition that may be seen in clients who are experiencing short term but severe disorders or stressors such as a major injury or surgery. Clinical signs of this disorder include fatigue, apathy, edema, decreased serum protein, mild weight loss, muscle weakness, and wasting. (Page 1089)
    Cachexia--a type of hospital related protein calorie malnutrition that occurs in a client who has been hospitalized for prolonged periods of time. It develops gradually due to the client receiving an insufficient quantity of a nutritionally complete diet. The client ends up with a syndrome of emaciation, tissue wasting, severe underweight, and diarrhea. (Page 1089)
    Anorexia nervosa--self imposed starvation. Occurs primarily in adolescent and young adult females but is also seen in women in their middle years. People with anorexia do not lose their appetite but rigorously control intake. The typical person could be described as a perfectionist, achievement oriented, who seeks

control over her life by refusing to eat. Despite extreme emaciation, the disturbed body image of the person with anorexia nervosa will cause her to believe that she is too fat. (Page 1091)

Bulimia--characterized by a behavior pattern of uncontrollable binge eating of enormous amounts of food, followed by self-induced vomiting and use of laxatives or diuretics to control weight. Bulimics maintain a thin image, which makes the disorder difficult to detect. Tooth decay, menstrual irregularities, and severe electrolyte imbalance leading to life threatening cardiac arrhythmias are most common. (Page 1091)

Obesity--a body weight of 20 to 30 percent or more above the ideal weight. (Page 1090)

6. Questions to be included in the nutritional assessment regarding diet include: write down everything you have eaten or drunk in the last 24 hours. Is this a typical diet? Do you have regular meal times? Is your eating pattern the same at work as it is at home? Under what conditions do you usually eat? What foods do you especially like, and dislike? Areas of importance during the nutritional examination include: measurements (height, weight) and anthropometric indicators. (Page 1093-1094)

7. A general etiology related to Altered Nutrition: More than Body Requirements is excessive intake relative to metabolic need. Risk factors for excess caloric intake relative to metabolic need include low energy expenditure (for example, a sedentary life style), a hypometabolic state that may occur in certain diseases such as hypothyroidism, and large food intake due to compulsive eating, overfeeding, or social factors. (Page 1100)

8. Some practical advice for reducing food expenditures and the effort required for meal preparation for older couples include: buy only a few pieces of fruit at a time, one ripe, one medium, one green; buy only what you can see; make one-dish meals and save half; when making a favorite dish, make enough to freeze; and divide loaves of bread and keep half in the freezer. (Page 1106)

9. Strategies to help improve his appetite include: adding nutritional supplements; teaching about food; encouraging exercise; assisting with menu selection; preparing his tray to be attractive; positioning him comfortably to eat, and providing company while he eats. (Page 1106)

   A regular diet is used for clients requiring no particular medication; a soft diet may be used in the transition phase from a liquid diet to a regular diet; a liquid diet may be full or clear. A full liquid diet is used before and after surgery in infectious diseases and where chewing and swallowing are problems. Clear liquid is also used before and after surgery or when the illness is acute. (Page 1108)

10. Nursing strategies to maximize the client's nutritional status after abdominal surgery include encouraging new eating patterns that will be of benefit, close follow-up and counseling, and referral to support groups if appropriate. (Page 1127)

Self-Examination Questions

1. C

2. A

3. D

4. D

5. B

6. C

■ **CHAPTER 26**

Review Questions

1. The elimination history should focus on: the client's primary concern; her current understanding of the problem; her past experiences with this problem; and a review of the subjective manifestations, such as what she has been eating, her definition of diarrhea and vomiting, her usual diet, and any changes in her diet and fluid intake. (Page 1150)

2. Intake and output, weight, body surface area calculation, abdominal girth, and blood pressure   (Pages 1151-1152)

3. The examination should include general observation of the client for indications that the elimination process is altered or at risk. Observe: overall appearance, general movement, facial expression, posture, skin and mucous membranes, mental status. (Page 1152)

4. Additional data should describe the condition of the skin, abdomen, genitalia, perineal area, and urine and feces. If problems with mobility or orientation are observed, a mobility and neurological assessment is indicated. (Page 1153)

5. Colonic constipation (Page 1153)

6. Inadequate fluid intake; inadequate fiber intake; lack of availability of certain foods; change in daily routine; stress; lack of privacy; metabolic problems; little social support; chronic use of medications and/or enemas (Page 1153)

7. Determine Joe's usual elimination pattern and document incontinent episodes; collaborate with Joe regarding the best time to initiate bowel control measures; obtain an order for an oral stool softener if necessary to facilitate defecation; assess what fluids normally stimulate defecation for Joe and administer these before the time for bowel evacuation; provide assistance to the bathroom; maintain privacy and limit evacuation time to 15 to 20 minutes; instruct Joe to lean forward at the hips while sitting on the toilet, place hands over abdomen and apply manual pressure; provide acceptance and encouragement; collaborate with Joe to develop and carry out an exercise program; emphasize the importance of regular mealtimes and adequate fluids and fiber; and work together to develop a plan. (Page 1209)

8. Emphasize the importance of clean equipment, proper handwashing, and thorough washing of the scrotum and penis before inserting the catheter; discuss techniques and the rationale for lubricating the catheter adequately; demonstrate methods for correctly identifying the urinary meatus; explain how far to insert the catheter; provide a list of signs and symptoms of urinary tract infection. (Page 1210)

9. The results of the bowel and bladder training program should be evaluated according to the outcomes that were described and accepted by the nurse and the client. The progress should be documented in the client's record. If expected outcomes do not occur, reassessment and additional plans are necessary. Joe will probably find talking about urination and defecation embarrassing and unpleasant. A nurse who demonstrates a concerned approach can develop his trust and enhance his willingness to collaborate in the program.   The result will be greater autonomy. (Pages 1210-1211)

Self-Examination Questions

1. (1) T,   (2) F,   (3) T,   (4) T,   (5) F

2. (1) c, (2) e, (3) a, (4) b (5) d

3. Less than adequate fluid intake, less than adequate dietary intake, less than adequate fiber, immobility, lack of privacy, stress, chronic use of enemas and/or laxatives, change in daily routine

4. C

5. Client teaching

6. Stimulates peristalsis

■ CHAPTER 27

Review Questions

1. A. Ventilation: moving air into and out of the lungs
   B. Diffusion: the process of gas exchange between alveoli capillaries and between capillaries and tissues
   C. Perfusion: delivery of blood to the body for cellular gas exchange (Page 1216)

2. Life-style factors that affect oxygenation in healthy individuals include: fitness (exercise, conditioning), nutrition (weight, nutrient intake), smoking, substance abuse, and emotional stress. (Page 1225)

3. Differences in anatomy and physiology related to oxygenation in older persons include: connective tissue changes that cause some loss of lung elasticity; postural changes related to osteoporosis that decrease the capacity for lung expansion; a gradual decline in normal PO_2, which increases cardiac workload and reduces exercise tolerance. (Page 1227)

4. Hyperventilation: more air moves through the lungs than normal. Assessed by a low PCO_2 it cannot be assessed by watching the client breathe.
   Hypoventilation: inadequate movement of air into and out of the lungs. Detected by a rise in PCO_2, it cannot be accurately assessed by watching a person breathe. Signs and symptoms include: alterations in respirations, dyspnea, orthopnea, tachycardia, anxiety, and neurological changes such as altered judgment, coordination or level of consciousness. (Page 1228)

5. Hypoxia: lack of oxygen at the tissue level
   Hypercapnia: retention of CO_2
   Tissue necrosis: tissue death due to low oxygenation (Page 1230)

6. Oxygenation history: primary concern; current understanding; past health experiences; personal, family, and social history; subjective manifestations (Page 1231)

7. 1 pack per day x 24 years = 24 pack-years
   2 packs per day x 2 years = 4 pack-years
   Total: 24 pack-years + 4 pack-years = 28 pack-years (Page 1233)

   The role of the nurse with Mrs. Jones is preventive care, which includes education and screening. (Page 1250)

8. Teach Mr. King leg exercises to enhance venous return, breathing exercises to maximize lung expansion, and effective coughing to maintain airway patency. (Page 1255)

9. Nursing actions that will reduce oxygen demands include reducing activity, relieving anxiety, alleviating pain, and lowering body temperature. (Page 1262)

    The nurse's responsibility during oxygen therapy includes: post a "no smoking" sign; explain to client and family the significance of "no smoking" during oxygen therapy and show them the location and correct use of fire extinguishers; help the client store personal effects that might support combustion; make sure hospital equipment is grounded; remove volatile and petroleum-based products from the room. (Page 1296)

10. A client education program for Mr. Su should include information about: the pathophysiological process of his condition, his medications, signs and symptoms that indicate changes in his physiological status, and changes in his daily routine that can prevent further complications (for example, the need for fluids, the need to avoid caffeine drinks and measures to promote circulation, such as elastic stockings, exercise and walking). (Page 1311)

Self-Examination Questions

1. B

2. A

3. D

4. D

5. C

6. (1) e, (2) c, (3) d, (4) a, (5) b

■ **CHAPTER 28**

Review Questions

1. Non-rapid eye movement (NREM) sleep is defined as the period of sleep during which no eye movements can be observed and the eyelids are still. REM sleep includes several stages: Stage I: Light, lasts a few minutes. Vital signs and metabolic rate decrease, and the individual is easily aroused. Stage II: 5-10 minutes of relaxed sleep. Individual can be easily awakened. Stages III and IV: 15-30 minutes of deep sleep. The individual is not disturbed by sensory stimuli; there is loss of muscle tone, reflexes are diminished, and snoring may occur. Stage IV sleep rests, relaxes, and physically restores the body. During NREM sleep the body repairs tissue and conserves energy. (Pages 1319-1320)

    After about 90 minutes of sleep, the individual returns from stage IV to stage I. Instead of awakening, the individual enters REM (rapid eye movement) sleep. Rapid eye movements, dreams, muscular twitching, and profound muscle relaxation occur. The sleeper is awakened with difficulty. At the completion of REM sleep, the individual descends through stages II to IV. Everyone averages 4-5 sleep cycles, each lasting 95-100 minutes per night. Stage IV sleep decreases and REM sleep increases with each cycle. When awakened during any stage of this cycle, the individual must resume sleep at Stage I and progress through the stages to REM sleep. REM sleep restores one mentally, provides a review of the day's events, and allows information to be categorized and stored for later retrieval. (Page 1320)

2. Irritability, increased sensitivity to pain, apathy, lack of alertness (Page 1320)

3. Age, environment, diet, stress, exercise, illness, medications, alcohol and stimulants, pain and discomfort (Pages 1321-1322)

4. Sleep apnea, narcolepsy (Page 1324)

5. Sleep walking, enuresis, confusional arousal (Page 1324)

6. Anxiety over finances, living arrangement or health; depression related to isolation, loneliness, or grief; physical discomfort due to pain, respiratory problems, or the environment (excessive heat, cold, or noise); acute confusion; sundown syndrome (Page 1324)

7. A. Physical: Activity intolerance, diarrhea
    B. Emotional: Anxiety, grieving
    C. Self-conceptual: Disturbed self-esteem, hopelessness
    D. Sociocultural: Ineffective coping, social isolation
    E. Sexual: Altered sexuality patterns, sexual dysfunction (Page 1329)

8. A. Primary concern directly or indirectly related to sleep
    B. Current understanding of how primary causes may affect sleep
    C. Past health problems/experiences
    D. Personal, family, and social history
    E. Subjective manifestations (Pages 1325-1327)

9. A. Teach the client progressive relaxation.
    B. Suggest limiting evening fluid intake, especially beverages with caffeine and alcohol.
    C. Suggest a warm bath before bedtime.
    D. Consult with physician regarding an analgesic to be given before bedtime. (Pages 1332-1333)

10. A. Disorders in initiating and maintaining sleep
    B. Disorders of excessive somnolence
    C. Disorders of arousal (Pages 1322-1324)

Self-Examination Questions

1. D

2. C

3. D

4. A

5. C

6. Anxiety over impending adulthood, family problems, sexual problems, drug abuse, alcohol abuse, menstrual problems, thyroid problems, and irregular sleep wake problems

7. Sleepwalking, sleeptalking, confusional arousals, enuresis

■ **CHAPTER 29**

Review Questions

1. Reception, perception, and response (Page 1351)

2. Immediate memory, short-term memory, long-term memory (Page 1353)

3. Genetic heritage, age, diet, environment, psychosocial factors, medications and other substances (Pages 1359-1361)

4. Alert: fully aroused and fully oriented to person, place, and time
    Confused: difficulty correctly interpreting and attending to stimuli; needs help to focus; disoriented to time, place, and person
    Delirious: restless, incoherent, agitated; alterations in thought processes
    Obtunded: sleeping or drowsy but arouses easily
    Stuporous: usually lethargic, slow to arouse, and drowsy
    Semi-consciousness: unresponsive, does not move spontaneously unless a noxious stimulus is applied
    Coma: state of unarousability to deep noxious stimuli
    Deep coma: completely unresponsive; lacks any response to deep noxious stimuli, lacks corneal, pupillary, gag, tendon, and plantar reflexes (Page 1362)

5. Can the client see and hear adequately?
    Does the client have the balance necessary for safe ambulation?
    Is the client's judgment adequate for safe performance of activities of daily living?
    Can the client communicate sufficiently to make needs known?
    Does the client have the coordination necessary for bathing and eating? (Page 1370)

6. The Glascow Coma Scale is a simple, consistent guide for grading level of consciousness. It focuses on cognitive behaviors and measures eye opening, motor response, and verbal response. (Page 1378)

7. Seat belt usage, driving without consumption of alcohol, using car lights when it becomes dark driving. (Page 1387)

8. Proper lighting, adequate night lights, large-print reading material, eyeglasses (Page 1389)

9. Determine whether there were any warning signs; assess where the seizure began and how it proceeded; note type of body movements; note change in size of pupils; determine the duration of the seizure and phases; describe the behavior after the seizure; note any weakness or paralysis of extremities after the seizure; note lethargy and amount of sleep required after the seizure. (Page 1406)

10. Analgesics; medical treatment; and noninvasive treatments such as relaxation, biofeedback, and imagery (Pages 1410-1411)

Self-Examination Questions

1. Arousal corresponds to wakefulness--a state of attention to people, things, and events in the environment. Without arousal, awareness is impossible. Content is what is contained in the conscious mind--the awareness of thoughts, sensations, and feelings.

2. C

3. Immediate memory, short-term memory, long-term memory. Short-term memory holds items for several minutes to hours.

4. Comprehension, reasoning, problem solving, judgment, and concept formation.

5. Speech is the mechanism for the production of verbal expression and encompasses the articulatory aspect of communication. Language is the assignment of a series of sounds, signs, gestures, or marks to designate and refer to objects, persons, and concepts. Language is used as the content of speech.

6. Establish pain onset, duration, location, intensity, and quality.

7. <u>Spasticity</u> is a state of hypertonic muscle tone in which the muscle responds with extreme resistance upon passive lengthening. <u>Flaccidity</u> is a state in which muscle tone is hypotonic, and the muscle is soft and floppy, offering no resistance upon passive lengthening. <u>Rigidity</u> is a state of constant resistance to movement.

■ **CHAPTER 30**

Review Questions

1. Body composition, strength flexibility, endurance (Pages 1422-1423)

2. Age, disability, health status, self-concept and emotions, values and beliefs, life-style (Pages 1425-1426)

3. Aerobic exercise: causes a sustained increase in heart rate and stroke volume and leads to improved oxygen use by muscles (Page 1423)
    Valsalva maneuver: attempting a forced expiration with the glottis closed; no movement of air occurs, but intrathoracic pressure increases, thereby decreasing blood flow in the major thoracic and coronary blood vessels (Page 1428)
    Isotonic exercise: exercise in which the tension within the muscles remains constant as its length changes to move resistance through a range of motion (Page 1422)
    Isometric exercise: involves near maximal contractions against a fixed object; the length of the muscle does not change because there is no joint movement during the contraction. (Pages 1422-1423)
    Orthostatic hypotension: a precipitous drop in blood pressure associated with standing; When an active individual rises from a recumbent position, reflex vasoconstriction of peripheral arterioles maintains blood pressure and blood supply to the brain. This reflex is dulled with bed rest. Therefore, vessels remain dilated, blood pools in the legs, and central blood pressure falls. (Page 1428)
    Active range of motion exercises: isotonic exercises (Page 1471)
    Activities of daily living (ADL): self-care skills required for independent living, including hygiene, grooming, and dressing (Page 1486)

4. Clients whose spontaneous movements are greatly decreased (unconscious, paralyzed, heavily sedated, elderly); obese clients, whose increased weight and dense subcutaneous tissue creates greater external pressure on capillaries over bony prominences; clients with edema; poorly nourished clients; clients who are incontinent; clients favoring Fowler's position (Page 1429)

5. Age; usual activity level; duration of activity reduction; weight; reclining/standing blood pressure; reclining/standing pulse, including rhythm strength; resting respirations, including rhythm, depth, quality; joint ROM, muscle strength, neurological status, health history (Page 1455)

6. Paralysis, mechanical or prescribed immobilization, severe pain, altered level of consciousness (Page 1427)

7. Establish a baseline; use the baseline and goals to prescribe exercise and activities; dispel misconceptions about exercise; discuss obstacles to exercise and strategies to overcome them; emphasize the value of play; provide feedback and positive reinforcement; be a good role model. (Pages 1463-1464)

8. Start with correct posture; maintain a wide base of support; use large muscles; use your body as a counterweight; minimize friction; incorporate leverage when possible. (Pages 1467-1468)

9. Footboard, individual foot supports, bed cradle, trochanter roll, sheepskin, hand roll, special bed and mattress, such as a pressure relief bed (Pages 1526-1527)

10. Federal legislation on the use of restraints (OBRA--the Omnibus Budget Reconciliation Act of 1987) became effective in October 1990. It ensures the right of all residents of nursing home facilities to be free from physical or pharmacological restraints unless they represent a specific treatment for a diagnosed condition. It also guarantees the right to refuse to be restrained. Under this law, nursing homes may be found liable for using restraints for staff convenience or in place of surveillance. The law does not currently apply to acute care facilities. Nurses need to consider the emotional impact of restraints on clients and their families, the effect on a client's self-concept, and physical and legal ramifications. Nurses must identify high-risk populations, make environmental modifications, individualize care, provide assistance with elimination, and educate staff. (Page 1531)

Self-Examination Questions

1. D

2. C

3. B

4. B

5. A

■ **CHAPTER 31**

Review Questions

1. Common functions of body fluids include: dispersal of and regulation of body temperature; transport of nutrients to cells; transport of waste products away from cells; transport of hormones to activity sites; lubrication of joint spaces; and maintenance of hydrostatic pressure in the cardiovascular system. (Page 1546)

2. Factors that affect fluid and electrolyte balance include: age, climate, stress, diet, illness, medications, and medical treatments. (Pages 1557-1560)

3. hyponatremia (sodium deficit)--signs and symptoms: dizziness, vertigo, hypotension; causes: GI fluid loss, increased sweat loss, diuretic abuse, adrenal insufficiency
    hypernatremia (sodium excess)--signs and symptoms: thirst, fever, dry sticky mucous membranes, confusion, headaches; causes: heat stroke, diarrhea, increased insensible loss, diabetes insipidus, excess infusion of hypertonic or isotonic saline
    hypokalemia (potassium deficit)--signs and symptoms: muscle weakness, cardiac arrhythmias, abdominal distension, depressed tendon reflexes; causes: diarrhea, gastric suction, diuretic use, metabolic alkalosis, poor intake

hyperkalemia (potassium excess)--signs and symptoms: irritability, anxiety, muscular weakness, cardiac irregularities, nausea and vomiting; causes: renal failure, RBC hemolysis, tissue trauma, metabolic acidosis, transfusion of blood, potassium sparing diuretics

hypocalcemia (calcium deficit)--signs and symptoms: muscle tetany, spasm, abnormal burning, bradycardia, hypotension, respiratory spasms; causes: decreased intake, insufficient vitamin D, severe diarrhea, burns

hypercalcemia (calcium excess)--signs and symptoms: bone and joint pain, lethargy, anorexia, muscle weakness; causes: increased PTH release, breast and lung cancers, prolonged immobilization

hypomagnesemia (magnesium deficit)--signs and symptoms: muscle spasticity, cardia arrhythmias, muscle tetany; causes: chronic alcohol abuse, diuretic abuse, malnutrition, diarrhea

hypermagnesemia (magnesium excess)--signs and symptoms: respiratory depression, lethargy, bradycardia, depressed reflexes; causes: renal failure, excess antacid, laxative use

hypophosphatemia (phosphate deficit)--signs and symptoms: nausea and vomiting, anorexia, bone destruction; causes: diabetic ketoacidosis, malabsorption states, low PO_4^-

hyperphosphatemia (phosphate excess)--signs and symptoms: muscle tetany, muscle weakness; causes: decreased excretion of PO_4^- , lack of PTH

hypochloremia (chloride deficit)--signs and symptoms: irritability, hypotension, lethargy, tachycardia; causes: vomiting, GI suction, diuretic use, diaphoresis

hyperchloremia (chloride excess)--signs and symptoms: weakness, lethargy, deep, rapid breathing; causes: severe dehydration, head injury, steroid use (Page 1564)

4. A. Respiratory depression as a result of narcotic overdose: respiratory acidosis
    B. Hyperventilation from anxiety: respiratory alkalosis
    C. Renal failure: metabolic acidosis
    D. Excessive gastric suction: metabolic alkalosis (Page 1566)

5. The most common observations associated with body fluid assessment include: mental status, facial expression, appearance, and speech. (Page 1570)

6. A. Apathy, restlessness, apprehension: electrolyte imbalance, especially hypernatremia, hyperkalemia, and hypercalcemia
    B. Dry, sticky mucous membranes: fluid volume deficit, hypernatremia
    C. Erythema and swelling of the tongue: hypernatremia
    D. Crackles on auscultation: fluid volume excess
    E. Ascites: plasma to interstitial fluid shift, liver disease, starvation diet
    F. Increased urine output: diuretic abuse, diabetes insipidus, hyperglycemia, hypoaldosteronism
    G. Hyperactive deep tendon reflexes: hypocalcemia
    H. Muscle flaccidity: hyperkalemia. (Page 1575)

7. Risk factors for fluid volume deficit include: extremes of age; excessive fluid loss through normal routes, e.g., vomiting, diarrhea, and diuretic use; excessive fluid loss through abnormal routes, e.g., indwelling tubes and urinary and small bowel diversions; deviations affecting access to intake and/or absorption of fluid; factors influencing fluid needs, e.g., hypermetabolic states; and knowledge deficit related to fluid volume. (Pages 1578-1581)

8. Strategies for identifying clients at risk for fluid imbalances include: health screening; life-style counseling; values clarification; and health education. (Page 1582)

9. The nurse's role in treating fluid and electrolyte imbalances includes: diet and fluid counseling; oral dehydration; oral electrolyte intake; limitation of oral fluid intake; limitation or oral electrolyte intake; and intake and output monitoring and recording. (Pages 1586-1587)

10. The nurse's responsibility includes: preventing metabolic complications, e.g., monitoring glucose levels to detect hyperglycemia, osmotic excesses, or fluid shifts; preventing apparatus complications, e.g., signs and symptoms of inflammation at the catheter site. (Pages 1622-1623)

Self-Examination Questions

1. A

2. C

3. C

4. C

5. A

6. A

■ **CHAPTER 32**

Review Questions

1. Science is a form of discovery, the basic aim of which is to explain natural phenomena. In science, explanations are called theories. Thus, science is an organized body of knowledge in the form of theories, and a process. It is important for nurses to understand the nature of science as it relates to nursing because nurses are vital to advancing nursing science through identification of knowledge for practice, evaluation of research for scientific merit, application of research findings in practice, generation of important research questions, and collaboration to produce research studies for the betterment of nursing care. (Page 1631)

2. The ways nurses can know if available nursing knowledge is adequate to guide nursing action, using Pierce's method of knowing, are through tenacity, authority, intuition, and science. Although all four methods rely on experience and contain a way to add knowledge over time, only science has self-correcting features. None of these methods is fail-proof, but because science attempts to find and expose its own errors, it can yield the more dependable and transmittable knowledge base for nursing practice. (Page 1630)

3. Phenomenon: the thing or event that attracts the scientist's attention
   Concept: a label applied to the sensory data that tells the scientist the phenomenon is occurring
   Theory: a statement or set of statements that aims to describe, explain, predict, or control a phenomenon
   Validity: the extent to which an instrument measures what it is designed to measure
   Reliability: the extent to which repeated measurements, using an instrument under stable conditions, yield the
        same results (Pages 1631-1633)

4. Descriptive theories describe the features of a phenomena common to multiple occurrences of it; explanatory theories relate two or more concepts; predictive theories stipulate which concepts are causes and which are effects. (Page 1633)

5. Stating the research question; developing the research problem; reviewing related research; forming hypotheses and defining variables; designing the research study; selecting the sample; collecting the data; analyzing the data; interpreting and communicating results; protecting human subjects in research (Page 1634)

6. Exploratory--a flexible research plan unique to the particular situation being investigated and allowing the researcher to explore new clues as they present themselves. Assuring reliability and minimizing bias are key considerations.

    Descriptive--a structured research plan that allows phenomena to be studied under naturally occurring conditions. Key features of descriptive designs include a conceptual and operational definition of variables, systematic sampling procedures, valid and reliable instrumentation, and data collection procedures that achieve some environmental control.

    Correlational--a structured plan that allows the study of relationships between two or more variables. A key feature of correlation studies is a sample that represents the population of interest and contains the full range of possible values for the variables of interest.

    Quasi-experimental--a structured plan that permits the limited study of causes and effects. Key features of quasi-experiments are nonequivalent control groups or repeated measures over time.

    Experimental--a structured research plan that permits the study of causes and effects. Key features of experiments are manipulation of the independent variable, control of the experimental situation, use of a control group, and random assignment of subjects to groups. (Page 1636)

7. Quantitative research is not inherently superior to qualitative research. Qualitative research methods yield data that are more narrative than numerical. Data are analyzed by the techniques of coding, sorting, and grouping. Quantitative research yields numerical data. Data are analyzed using statistical techniques. Studies using quantitative methods result in numerical descriptions or test hypotheses. These two types of research methods are the methods used most often in nursing research and are necessary to allow nurses to study concepts of interest to nurses. (Page 1640)

8. Four commonly used nursing conceptual frameworks are King's theory of goal attainment, Orem's self-care deficit theory, Roy's adaptation model, and Roger's science of unitary human beings model.

    King's basic thesis is that a client and nurse perceive each other and their situation, share information, state goals related to the client's health, explore means, and act to attain goals. This interactive process uses a set of three interlocking systems: personal, interpersonal, and social. (Page 1641)

    The main thesis in Orem's model is that people require nursing care when their needs for care exceed their ability to meet these needs. Orem calls needs "self-care requisites" and ability the "self-care agency" When needs exceed ability, the situation is called a "self-care deficit." (Page 1642)

    The basic thesis of the Roy model is that nurses promote clients' adjustments to challenges that they encounter in that dimension of life relating to health and illness. To Roy, adjusting is called "adaptation" and challenges are called "stimuli." (Page 1644)

    Rogers' proposed a highly abstract conceptual model using terms not ordinarily applied to people. The central thesis of her model is that people and their environment are integrated and that their mutual interaction produces the unfolding of a person's life process of development. The role of nurses is to support this process by promoting a harmonious interaction of person and environment and strengthening the integrity of each. (Page 1645)

9. Clinical observation method, survey method, cross-sectional method, retrospective method, longitudinal method, experimental method (Page 1648)

10. A. Identifying knowledge for practice
    B. Evaluating the scientific merit of research studies
    C. Applying knowledge in practice
    D. Raising research questions
    E. Collaborating to produce research (Pages 1651-1655)

Self-Examination Questions

1. Person, environment, health, nursing

2. Descriptive, explanatory, predictive

3. Protection from harm; full disclosure; freedom to participate or not; privacy and confidentiality; protection of vulnerable subjects

4. (1) g, (2) e, (3) a, (4) b, (5) d, (6) f, (7) c

5. (1) d, (2) a, (3) b, (4) c

6. a, c, e, f

■ **CHAPTER 33**

Review Questions

1. A. Asking questions that gather information about the meaning of life experiences to clients. For example, did a client have enough information to make an informed consent? Was a certain procedure or treatment necessary? Were there other options that could have been discussed with the client?

   B. Examining the validity of claims and client's beliefs and knowledge to determine whether this information is true or false. For example, just because a neighbor or close relative had a negative experience or prognosis with cancer does not mean that this client also will.

   C. Providing philosophic arguments (good reasons for communicating clients' requests to others for action). For example, assisting the client to voice concerns about a specific upcoming test or procedure to the physician. (Pages 1660-1661)

2. Empiricism, the basis for the scientific method, states that knowledge of the world is most reliable and best achieved by observation through the senses. For example, regular handwashing contributes to decreasing infection rates. (Page 1662)
   Rationalism attempts to find a basis for knowledge through reasoning alone. It does this by questioning beliefs and propositions developed from everyday experiences. For example, does a nurse who commits multiple medication errors have a drug abuse problem? (Page 1663)

3. Epistemology studies the knowledge questions of philosophy. It is concerned with how knowledge is achieved and how accurate it is. For example, what knowledge does the client need to make an informed choice regarding two different methods or approaches to cancer treatment? Epistemology can be a useful tool for nurses to use in questioning current nursing ideas and practices as well as in developing and critiqueing nursing research. (Page 1664)

4. Metaphysical questions about identity and change, mind and body, and free will and determination all can have a bearing on nursing practice. For example, is the woman in the nursing home the same person she was when she was middle aged (identity and change)? How do illness and disability affect a person's body image (mind and body)? Is it always the role of the client to get well (free will and determination)? (Page 1665)

5. Ethics is the branch of philosophy that analyzes the morality of the decisions nurses make. (Page 1666)

6. Key assumptions of the mutual interaction model include genuine respect for client personhood, sharing of the nurse-client perspectives, and client autonomy (self-direction in all clinical decisions). (Page 1670)

7. Case A. 1. Substituted judgement includes evidence in the medical record such as a health care proxy; do-not-resuscitate orders; surrogate family decision maker, conservator, or guardian; and living will. 2. The best standard of care measures consider direct care decisions in terms of benefits for the client, such as reducing discomfort, avoiding harm, and improving quality of life. (Page 1671)

   Case B. Helping the client to discuss other care options with the physician, such as a hospice (sharing of prospective and respect for client autonomy). (Page 1671)

8. (1) d, (2) c, (3) a, (4) b (Page 1666)

9. In some client situations it will be more important for the nurse to provide a caring response rather than continuing to give care which may not help, for example, continuing to give antibiotics or dialysis to the permanently unconscious client. In such an instance, the most appropriate response may be for the nurse to advocate with the physicians and family that such treatment be stopped. (Page 1670)

10. Answers will vary.

Self-Examination Questions

1. (1) e, (2) g, (3) i, (4) f, (5) a, (6) h, (7) b, (8) c, (9) d, (10) j

2. (1) empiricist; (2) thinking, reason, or rationality; (3) identity and change; (4) free will; (5) mind-body problem; (6) holism; (7) caring; (8) participate in care, accept consequences of choices

3. (1) b, (2) c, (3) a

4. (1) F, (2) T   (3) F, (4) T, (5) F, (6) T, (7) T,   (8) F,   (9) F, (10) T

5. C

6. C

■ **CHAPTER 34**

Review Questions

1. Ethics, a branch of philosophy, is concerned with the principles and theories that promote right or best actions within a given situation. (Page 1677)

2. An ethical problem is a situation in which the right or good thing to do is clear, but accomplishing it is very difficult. An ethical dilemma is a situation in which two or more alternatives for action will have undesirable consequences. (Page 1678)

3. A. Choosing one's beliefs and behaviors
   B. Prizing one's beliefs and behaviors
   C. Acting on one's beliefs (Page 1678)

4. A. Choosing from alternatives
    B. Considering consequences
    C. Choosing freely
    D. Being proud of and cherishing
    E. Publicly affirming
    F. Acting on
    G. Acting consistently or with a pattern (Page 1678)

5. A. Respect of person (unconditional dignity and worth of each person)
    B. Respect of autonomy (self-determination of choices)
    C. Nonmaleficence (duty to do no harm)
    D. Beneficence (duty to do good)
    E. Justice (fair distribution of scarce resources)
    F. Fidelity (keeping promises)
    G. Confidentiality (individual's right to privacy)
    H. Veracity (devotion to the truth) (Pages 1685-1689)

6. Teleology holds that good or right actions are measured by the consequences of those actions in relation to either the benefits for the most individuals (act-utilitarianism) or the moral rules of society (rule-utilitarianism).

    Deontology holds that a person ought to carry out certain duties or actions without regard to consequences. For example, a nurse should inform a client that surgery causes postoperative pain even though she or he may not like to do this and the client may not like to hear it. (Page 1690)

7. (1) b, (2) c, (3) a, (4) d (Page 1684)

8. self-determination, health, caring, client advocacy (Page 1684)

9. Paternalism can be justified when a client is: not capable of making sound judgment in a particular instance; in probable danger of doing serious harm to himself or another; or likely to agree at a later time that paternalistic action was justified. (Page 1693)

10. (1) f, (2) e, (3) c, (4) b, (5) g, (6) a, (7) d (Page 1697)

Self-Examination Questions

1. An example of an ethical dilemma could be any expression of two ethical principles in tension, such as autonomy versus nonmaleficence; doing good versus avoiding harm; truth-telling versus avoiding harm; "whistle blowing" (truth-telling) versus loyalty.

2. Any five values from Tables 34-1 and 34-2 would be correct. Examples include: accountability, search for truth (research), collaboration, self-regulation, quality care.

3. (1) c, (2) g, (3) b, (4) f, (5) e, (6) a, (7) d, (8) h

4. D

5. A

6. The ability to understand choices; the ability to recognize and weigh risks and benefits; the ability to see choices in light of one's values and life plan; the freedom to act on these choices

7. Preservation of autonomy; avoidance of harm; likely ratification at a later time

8. Ethical principles

■ CHAPTER 35

Review Questions

1. It is important for nurses to have an understanding of the organizational structure of government and the roles played by government in facilitating and providing health care services because doing so will enable nurses to assist clients through the health care system. The nurse will frequently encounter clients who need assistance in obtaining and financing health care but who may not be aware of government services available to help them or how to gain access to those services. (Page 1702)

2. Federal--Health Care Financing Administration regulates the distribution of federal funds under Medicare and
        Medicaid. (Page 1702)
    State--State health departments have licensing responsibility for local health care facilities. (Page 1705)
    Local--control of infectious disease, management of school health programs, immunization plans (Page 1705)

3. Accreditation--a process wherein an institution seeks evaluation by an outside agency. State accreditation is
        usually a mandatory process. Schools of nursing must be state accredited. (Page 1708)
    Utilization review--evolved from the 1965 Social Security Act, which mandated that health care reimbursement
        under Medicare and Medicaid would be provided only for health care that was medically necessary. To
        implement this standard, legislation requires that each institution seeking federal reimbursement for health
        care establish a utilization committee. The committee was to review the necessity for client admissions,
        the reasons supporting length of hospital stay, and the appropriateness of the treatment provided. These
        reviews were retrospective, that is, they occurred after the care was given and billed. (Page 1708)
    Health maintenance organization--an organized system of health care delivery whose members prepay a monthly
        fee that is guaranteed to cover all services named in the contract. (Page 1710)
    Hospice care--a specific type of care designed for terminally ill clients who chose to spend their remaining
        days at home or in a homelike setting rather than in an institution. A hospice team assists clients and
        family members to cope with the dying process and the stages of grief and bereavement. (Page 1706)
    Case managers--assess clients' overall needs for different health services, delineate comprehensive client
        outcomes, identify and procure the most cost-effective means of meeting these outcomes, and evaluate the
        effectiveness of procured services. (Page 1717)

4. Fee for service--consumers pay for each health service as it is provided.
    Capitation--requires that individuals or employers pay a negotiated fee, which pays for a package of health care
        services during a specific time period.
    Fee for diagnosis--a type of prospective payment service in which facilities are given a fixed dollar amount
        for the treatment of a client before services are provided. The fee amount is based on the client's
        principal diagnosis, secondary diagnosis, demographic data such as age and sex, and usual treatment
        necessary for the client's health problem. (Page 1710)

5. The main sources of payment for care are: direct personal payment, private insurance payment, and government
    health plans. (Pages 1710-1711)

6. Medicare was designed to provide health care to individuals 65 years of age and older. It is organized into Part
    A and Part B. Part A is available to the disabled and to individuals age 65 and over who are eligible for
    Social Security or railroad retirement. It provides insurance toward hospitalization. Medicare clients pay a

deductible amount and have copayment responsibilities. Medicare Part B is voluntary. It provides partial coverage for physician services to those eligible for Part A coverage, on payment of a monthly premium.

Medicaid is a financial aid program designed to provide medical assistance to low income persons who are aged, disabled, blind, or members of families with dependent children. It is jointly sponsored by the federal and state government. The federal government established broad guidelines for the operation of the program and provides matching funds to states that meet the guidelines. (Pages 1711-1712)

7. Four of the circumstances that have led to the present problems in health care are: fragmented health care financing, changing patterns of health and disease, rising consumer expectations, and advances in technology. (Pages 1713-1716)

8. Price controls--the Omnibus Budget Reconciliation Act of 1990, for example, limits payment for hospital outpatient services and establishes a fee schedule for physician services based on the resource-based relative value scale.

Regulation of market services--sets prescriptions on quality of services, who may provide services, and who must receive services.

Competition--proposals to reduce restrictions on health care delivery and promote freemarket competition among providers and insurers was introduced with the expectation that competition would result in downward pressures on prices and greater efficiency in providing health care.

Alternative insurance delivery systems--such as HMOs can offer services at substantially lower premiums because they have more control over use of services of contracted providers.

Managed care--refers to plans that coordinate a broad range of client services and monitor care to assure that it is appropriate and provided in the most efficient and inexpensive way.

Alternative professional providers--including nurse practitioners, midwives, and clinical nurse specialists, whose services include physical assessment, diagnostic screening, and teaching as well as traditional health care treatment. (Pages 1716-1717)

9. Activities that community centers have developed to maximize individual wellness include adult day care centers, nutritional counseling, mental health services, and healthy social activities. (Page 1717)

10. The key features of nursing's agenda for health care reform include: enhanced access to care by delivering primary care in community based settings; emphasis on personal responsibility for individual health based on informed decision making; use of most cost-effective providers; and the Health Start Plan, which focuses on underserved, vulnerable populations. (Page 1719)

Self-Examination Questions

1. (1) a, (2) a, (3) a, (4) a, (5) b, (6) b, (7) c

2. False, false, true

3. True, true, false

4. a and b

5. (1) b, (2) c, (3) a

6. A

■ CHAPTER 36

Review Questions

1. Economics is the study of the efficient allocation of scarce resources. It is important for nurses to understand the importance of economics in health care. Increasingly, health care services are being evaluated for economic efficiency. Because nursing care is one of the largest components of health service, nurses must help improve the operating efficiency of the health care industry. As health professionals collaborate to maximize the health of society, nurses must lead in minimizing the use of resources while maximizing the resources. (Page 1726)

2. Efficiency: the amount of resources used to achieve a desired result (Page 1727)

   Productivity: a measure of efficiency with which labor, materials, and equipment are converted into goods and services (Page 1727)

   Effectiveness: concerned with results; it is a measure of whether the services provided have the intended or desired outcomes (Page 1727)

   Economic resources: refer to natural, man-made, or human resources used to produce material goods and services such as food, shelter, defense, and health care (Page 1726)

   Accountability: refers to the undertaking of practices to enable the tracking and explanation of the use of resources (Page 1728)

3. Two types of economic systems are capitalism and socialism. Capitalism applies to the political and economic system in which the market is allowed to determine resource allocation. Socialism disavows private ownership, competition, and profit. (Page 1729)

4. The basic components of the market system are: (1) a market; (2) economic exchanges that occur in a market; (3) producers; (4) consumers. (Page 1729)

5. The main characteristics of a competitive market are: (1) identical products are made by all producers; (2) perfect knowledge about alternative options is available to producers and consumers; therefore there are no uninformed decisions; (3) profits are maximized by producers and satisfaction is maximized by consumers; (4) there are enough buyers and sellers, acting independently, so that no one individual has a significant impact on prices; (5) there are no barriers to the entry and exit from the market of either producers or consumers. (Page 1730)

6. Demand and supply in the market interact to establish the price at which sellers offer just the amount that buyers wish to purchase. This is the point at which supply equals demand. (Page 1734)

7. Characteristics of the health care industry that interfere with market self correction are: fragmentation, relative consumer ignorance, selectivity in third-party payment, provider-agent conflict, skewed incentives, and infinite expendability. (Pages 1735-1736)

8. Six levels of economic decision making within the health care industry are: Level 1--how to maximize society's welfare; allocation of resources occur through health care policy; Level 2--industry responses to the social policy; allocation of resources within the health care system; Level 3--economic analysis by institutional leaders determines the most efficient combination of institutions and services to include within a multi-institutional system; allocation of resources within multi-institutional systems such as hospital chains; Level 4--single agencies must function within all the constraints established at the previous three levels; allocation of resources

within individual agencies and institutions; Level 5--the major focus is on determining the most efficient methods of providing services; allocation of resources within the departments of single institutions; Level 6--involve the priorities and practices of individual clinicians within a department. (Page 1738)

9. Six levels of economic decision making for nurses in the health care industry are: Level 1--nurses have a vital interest in the economic decisions made at the broad societal level (e.g., that all individuals have access to health services.); Level 2--nurses examine their health care objectives from an institutional perspective and consider the industry-wide impact of government policies and regulations on health care and nursing services; Level 3--nurses who work in multi-institutional systems are involved in setting policy for all facilities in the system; Level 4--nurses influence decisions on the optimal number of nursing staff, kinds of and amounts of services to be offered, and the combination of nursing personnel and supplies needed to produce them; Level 5--nurses make decisions about the direct provision of nursing services; Level 6--nurses make decisions about their priorities for providing direct client care. (Pages 1738-1740)

10. Individual nurses make economic decisions about their priorities for providing direct client care by: priority setting (e.g., how much time will be spent on notes or teaching a client); use of supplies (e.g., nurses decide which products to use); use of personnel (e.g., nurses are asking for computers to maximize their time with clients); economic collaboration with the client (e.g., nurses consider the client's wishes and values while planning care); clinical use of economic reasoning (e.g., nurses develop the mental habit of considering the benefits and costs of the clinical choices available). (Page 1740)

Self-Examination Questions

1. Every economic system (capitalist, socialist, communist) must decide (1) what goods and services are produced, (2) how the goods and services are produced, (3) how the goods and services are distributed, and (4) how much is consumed.

2. Fragmentation, relative consumer ignorance, selectivity in third-party payments, almost infinite expendability, skewed incentives in the provision of care, and provider-agent conflict

3. (1) Define the problem.
    (2) Generate alternative solutions.
    (3) Identify and quantify benefits and costs.
    (4) Compare benefits and costs.
    (5) Select the preferred alternative.
    (6) Monitor and reevaluate the conclusions reached.

4. In addition to price, the tastes and preferences of consumers, the number of buyers, the future expectations of those consumers, the prices of other goods and services, and the income of consumers, the demand for health care is determined by a need for the services, a recognition of that need, the availability of resources to obtain care, a motivation to seek care, and the services available.

5. Health care costs have risen rapidly in recent years, consuming an expanding amount of limited resources. Although health care cost increases have slowed, the health care industry continues to grow more rapidly than the general economy. Increasingly, the production of health care services is being evaluated on the basis of economic efficiency. This emphasis places pressure on the various health care providers in the production process to demonstrate that they can produce the desired services economically. Nurses, therefore, must be able to demonstrate the effects of their various procedures on client outcome and demonstrate that they can provide the required interventions economically.

■ CHAPTER 37

Review Questions

1. Health care as an economic transaction means that health care can be viewed as an act of exchange into which people enter for their mutual benefit and welfare. (Page 1746)

2. Consumerism: promotion of consumer interests; one meaning in the literature views consumerism as the organized reaction of individuals to the perceived or real inadequacies of sellers and their products, to the marketplace or market mechanisms, or to government services or consumer policies; another definition of consumerism views it as the direct, face-to-face challenges to sellers' claims that consumers make in their efforts to be discriminating buyers (Page 1750)

   Management by objectives: an approach that seeks to obtain subordinate commitment to employee performance objectives through participative goal-setting (Page 1772)

   Mutual interaction: model of professional interaction that combines collaborative aims with the decision-making framework of the nursing process (Page 1759)

   Shared governance: a democratic approach to the exercise of authority and control in an organization; involves participation by people at all levels of the organization in decisions about policy and use of resources (Page 1772)

   Transformational leadership: real changes initiated by a leadership process that carry through from decision-making stages to the point of concrete changes to peoples' lives, attitudes, behaviors, and institutions (Page 1774)

   Collaboration: a process in which two or more individuals work together jointly influencing one another for the attainment of a goal (Page 1759)

3. Problems in achieving distributive justice in health care are: increased cost of insurance; high cost of health care; many small businesses no longer provide health care benefits; erosion of Medicaid over the last few years; increase of out-of-pocket costs of Medicare; expected growth of long-term care due to an increase in the elderly population; financial base for Medicare is at risk service-shifting to health care centers and clinics; and a severe shortage of nurses. (Page 1746)

4. Alternatives to the current system include market proposals which limit the role of government; play or pay; national health insurance; and a Canadian-style system for the United States. (Pages 1748-1750)

5. The main aspects of the Consumer Bill of Rights are: the right to safety; the right to be informed; the right to choose; and the right to be heard. (Page 1751)

6. Phases in the mutual interaction model include: exploratory phase--initial contact between client and nurse; informational sharing and analysis--nurse and client clarify issues; mutual goal setting--determine with the client his or her developmental stage and the desired state to be achieved; strategy devising--nurse and client jointly select strategies to reach mutually define outcomes; implementation--strategy action is taken to meet client needs; evaluation--examine whether desired outcomes are met. (Pages 1760-1761)

7. Guidelines for negotiating and consensus building include: separate the person from the problem; separate the position from the person's interest; invent options for mutual gain; use objective decision criteria; focus attention on the merits. (Page 1766)

8. The management functions of nurse managers in health care agencies are planning, organizing, staffing, influencing, and controlling. (Page 1770)

9. Maslow: hierarchy of needs--a theory of motivation that indicates people are motivated by unsatisfied human needs, including physiological needs, safety, belonging, love, self esteem, and self-actualization
    McClelland: McClelland's trio--theory of motivation that relates motivation to a need for achievement, affiliation, and power
    Hertzberg: Hertzberg's factors--theory of motivation that relates motivation to satisfiers (elements that increase job satisfaction) and hygiene factors (Page 1771)

10. Four fundamental characteristics of leadership are: leadership is a relationship based on influence; the leadership relationship includes at least one leader and one follower; leaders and followers purposefully desire certain changes, and these changes must be of a transforming nature; the mutuality of purposes between leaders and followers is forged through their noncoercive influence relationship. (Page 1773)

Self-Examination Questions

1. B

2. Antiauthority trends; consumer education; growth of allied health professions; medical ethics

3. Determining health care wants/needs; making product/service comparisons; identifying the best value

4. C

5. D

6. A

7. Arguing positions is not the most efficient way to reach an agreement and may have the undesirable effect of damaging the nurse/client relationship.

8. Figurehead; public relations problem solver; liaison and networker; information conduit; spokesperson and chief communicator; resource handler and supervisor